Pregnancy Thrombophilia:
Key Concepts and Clinical Treatment

Pregnancy Thrombophilia: Key Concepts and Clinical Treatment

Edited by **Alex Bradley**

New Jersey

Published by Foster Academics,
61 Van Reypen Street,
Jersey City, NJ 07306, USA
www.fosteracademics.com

Pregnancy Thrombophilia: Key Concepts and Clinical Treatment
Edited by Alex Bradley

International Standard Book Number: 978-1-63242-328-3 (Hardback)

Printed in the United States of America.

Contents

Preface

Pregnancy thrombophilia poses serious challenges for both the mother and the fetus. This book helps the readers in learning the current observations regarding the effect and management of mother-fetal thrombophilia, the achievement required for gestation complication prevention and formulating an effective pregnancy valuation. It covers all the multi-faceted aspects of thrombophilic conditions during pregnancy, including basic and clinical knowledge approach. The book presents an account on the challenges and problems related to various aspects of pregnancy thrombophilia. Obstetricians, IVF experts, gynecologists, internists, and general practitioners, especially skilled in high risk pregnancy assessment will receive up to date evidence from this book regarding mother thrombophilia testing indications, an incoming pharmacogenetic approach of individualized antithrombotic therapy and thrombotic tendency management in assisted reproductive technics. Physicians, especially geneticists, biologists and researchers, who integrate the science of the laboratory with teaching practice, will derive essential benefits from discourses on physiological, pathological and molecular basis of maternal/fetus thrombophilia provided in the book. Also, mother-health incorporated immunologists will find a new therapeutic approach beyond anticoagulant treatment in pregnancy with autoimmune conditions from the book. It provides the readers with an opportunity for a quick review on current standpoints regarding maternal thrombotic state. It also provides them with authoritative and easy to read summary answers in the daily pregnancy follow up practice.

Various studies have approached the subject by analyzing it with a single perspective, but the present book provides diverse methodologies and techniques to address this field. This book contains theories and applications needed for understanding the subject from different perspectives. The aim is to keep the readers informed about the progress in the field; therefore, the contributions were carefully examined to compile novel researches by specialists from across the globe.

Indeed, the job of the editor is the most crucial and challenging in compiling all chapters into a single book. In the end, I would extend my sincere thanks to the chapter authors for their profound work. I am also thankful for the support provided by my family and colleagues during the compilation of this book.

Editor

Genetics and Molecular Pathophysiology of Thrombotic States

Ludek Slavik

Additional information is available at the end of the chapter

1. Introduction

Venous thrombosis is a multifactorial disease frequently related to the interaction of genetic and environmental risk factors. Testing for specific mutations in these patients helps to determine the decision on the duration of anticoagulant therapy, risk stratification for primary or secondary prophylaxis. Some of the recently discovered genetic risk factors, such as factor V Leiden and prothrombin G20210A mutations, are quite common in the population. When compared to functional assays, molecular assays provide clear results without different cut-off values. Accordingly, laboratory investigation of thrombophilic disorders has expanded due to incorporation of modern molecular assays. Criteria used to select specific DNA methodologies reflect the issues of cost, automation, speed, reliability, and simplicity for specific diagnostics. A variety of currently used molecular methods fulfill many, but not all of these criteria. The new methods of real-time PCR and DNA microarrays offer the potential for widespread application and utility in the future. Problems arise with interpretation in many new polymorphisms without significant clinical relevance.

Let's look at the history of molecular diagnosis of thrombophilia. Since the very beginning of the diagnosis of thrombophilic disorders, which arose from the study of families with a high frequency of thrombophilic complications, it was apparent that in a number of cases, the disorder was due to dominantly inherited conditions. Already the discovery of the first families presenting a defect in antithrombin (AT) led to the description of the genetic causes of this defect. As such, over 150 causes of AT mutation were described.

Molecular genetic methods were implemented into the screening examinations for thrombophilic disorders in the 1990's along with the first discoveries of coagulation inhibitors (AT, protein C and protein S). The discovery of the molecular cause of activated protein C (APC) resistance by Bertina in 1994 greatly expanded their utilization.

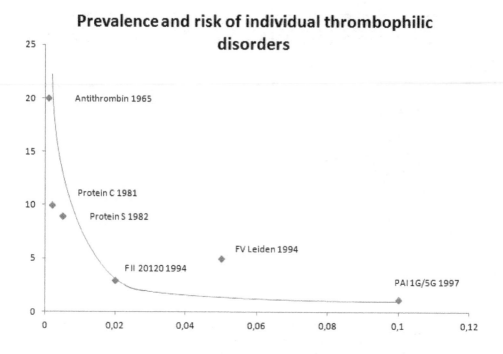

Figure 1. Prevalence and risk of individual thrombophilic markers with a time line representing their discovery[1] Despite the expansion of these methods, the following years brought forth discoveries of defects on a molecular basis, which posed decreasing risks of thrombosis, as can be seen in Fig 1. However, until the end of the last century, it has been assumed that further investigations of genetic causes of thrombophilia are needed to clarify the risk of this disorder in a more detailed manner. Currently, it is apparent that there is a deflection from this idea and attention is focused rather on the elucidation of the complex pathophysiology of coagulation at the molecular level.

Successive determination of relative risk of individual factors and their prevalence in the population led to the gradual definition of the panel of genetic thrombophilia. Currently, they can be divided into two groups i.e.1/ a well-defined genetic thrombophilic risk factors and 2/ potential risks factors of thrombophilia.Well-defined VTE risk factors include resistance to activated protein C (APCR) often due to factor V Leiden (FVL), prothrombin G20210A gene mutation (FII G20210A), high factor VIII (FVIII) activity or homocysteine level, and natural anticoagulant deficiencies: antithrombin (AT), protein C (PC), and protein S (PS). Patients with laboratory-confirmed thrombophilia are at greater risk for VTE, but most will never have such an event[2]. VTE risk increases synergistically as other risk conditions are acquired (eg, pregnancy, trauma, immobilization). More than 60% of patients with idiopathic (spontaneous or unprovoked) VTE have inherited thrombophilia[3].

An individual's risk for VTE would be determined by the combination of baseline propensity for thrombosis and the magnitude of the acute insult. In the face of genetically increased baseline hypercoagulability (major genetic thrombophilic state) even a relatively weak insult (e.g., blood stasis during a flight) can be sufficient to precipitate DVT. Likewise, in an individual with a relatively low level of baseline genetic hypercoagulability (potential genetic thrombophilic state) a relatively strong thrombogenic event (e.g., pregnancy) may be required to provoke an episode of VTE[4]. Thus, the precipitating event in such individuals is often clinically overt. In most cases, such thrombophilic individuals never suffer VTE throughout their lifetimes, and when they do have an episode, it is unlikely to recur. In contrast, an individual with a high level of baseline genetic hypercoagulability is at such high risk that relatively minor acquired triggers can initiate a thrombotic episode. These triggers are therefore subclinical, giving the appearance that the patient has "idiopathic", "spontaneous", or "unprovoked" VTE.

Thrombophilia	Prevalence* (%)	Relative risk
Antitrombin deficiency	0.02	10
Protein C deficiency	0.2 - 0.4	10
Protein S deficiency	< 1	10
FV Leiden (G1691A) homozygosity	0.02	50
FV Leiden (G1691A).heterozygosity	5-7	5 - 7
F II (G20210A)	2 - 7	2 - 3
Fibrinogen gamma 10034T	6	2

* prevalence in Caucasian population

Table 1. Prevalence and relative risk of venous thromboembolism associated with well defined major genetic risk factors[5]

2. Major genetic thrombophilic states

Major genetic thrombophilic states include defects with clinically confirmed risk for VTE and an understanding of the pathophysiological action of these defects.

2.1. Antithrombin

Egeberg first described familial antithrombin III deficiency, now termed antithrombin deficiency, in 1965[6]-[8]. This first work already pointed out that antithrombin deficiency is a significantly more serious risk factor for developing thrombosis than protein C and S deficiency, and that the majority of patients show clinical manifestation before the age of 25[7], [9]. This does not pertain to changes of the heparin binding site, which occurs frequently, and does not present a risk in the heterozygous form[9].

Based on extensive studies, the thrombotic risk for patients with AT deficiency was determined to be increased five-fold, based on the 1.1 % prevalcence of this deficiency in patients with venous thrombosis compared to 0.2 % prevalence in the control group[10]. Other studies determined the prevalence of AT deficiency to be between 1 – 0.5 % [6]. There are two primary types of antithrombin deficiency: type I and type II. Type I antithrombin deficiency is characterized by an inadequate amount of normal antithrombin present. In this case, there is simply not enough antithrombin present to inactivate the coagulation factors. In type II antithrombin deficiency, the amount of antithrombin present is normal, but it does not function properly and is thus unable to carry out its normal functions. In many cases, the antithrombin in type I deficiencies has a problem binding to heparin, although there have been multiple other changes to the antithrombin molecule described.

Antithrombin deficiency may be assessed by chromogenic or clotting laboratory methods. The chromogenic assay is the most simple and usually preferred. Overall, there are fewer confounders with antithrombin activity assays than with protein C or protein S activity assays; partly because chromogenic antithrombin activity assays are performed rather than clot-based[11]. For antithrombin activity, chromogenic (IIa- or Xa-) based assays which are not affected by heparin are available. Thrombin (IIa)-based assays, in theory, can be falsely elevated by elevated heparin cofactor II because heparin cofactor II is a natural inhibitor of thrombin. Factor Xa-based assays might be less sensitive to type II deficiencies than the IIa-based assays[12]. Direct thrombin inhibitors falsely increase results in IIa-based assays but not with Xa-based assays, because they inhibit factor IIa but not factor Xa[13].

A false-positive result for a type II deficiency may occur in the presence of a heparin-binding site (HBS) mutation. Extending the incubation time of the activity assay to 300 sec may help normalize results, since the extra time allows the assay to overcome this limitation and normalize results, whereas other (clinically important) mutations remain abnormal[14]. In general, HBS mutations are thought to be not significant except in homozygotes[14].

Another caveat with antithrombin testing involves different type II mutation called antithrombin Cambridge II A384S[15],[16]. Heterozygotes and homozygotes with this mutation were found to have normal activity in an anti-Xa assay (and appropriately low activity with an anti-IIa-based assay). Heterozygosity was found in 0.1–0.2% of the general population and 0.4–1.7% of patients with venous thrombosis. Heterozygosity was associated with a ninefold increased risk for venous thrombosis. The main disadvantage of screening for deficiency using an antithrombin antigen assays is that type II (qualitative) deficiencies will not be detected.

2.2. Protein C

The first studies demonstrating increased risk of thrombosis in patients with heterozygous protein C deficiency were presented in 1981[17],[18]. No difference between patients with various types of deficiency (I or II) and basic mutation were noted. These studies showed that a large majority of patients already has clinical manifestations of the disease at a young age[19]. In addition, it is interesting to note that in some patients, APC resistance was also present as an additional factor increasing the risk of thrombosis[20].

The prevalence of protein C deficiency in patients with venous thromboembolism has been determined to exist approximately 3%[21]-[23] compared to 0.2 % prevalence in the healthy population[18]. When compared with the control group, the relative thrombotic risk for protein C deficiency is apprixomately 6.5 fold[24]. Despite the relatively low population prevalence, the high risk of thrombogenicity results in a 1–2% contribution of protein C deficiency on all thrombophilic conditions.

Protein C deficiency can be detected by chromogenic or clotting methods. Both assays may have pitfalls in testing. Clot-based assays are aPTT- or Russell viper venom (RVV) based, either of which can give falsely high results in the presence of direct thrombin inhibitors. With aPTT-based assays, lupus anticoagulants can cause falsely high results and elevated factor VIII or factor V Leiden can cause falsely low results. Heterozygous factor V Leiden did not appear to affect an RVV-based assay, but artificially low protein C results in homozygous factor V Leiden patients could not be excluded due in part to the small number of such patients[25]. Lupus anticoagulants did not falsely increase protein C levels using an RVV-based assay[25], but according to the manufacturer, the possibility of lupus anticoagulant interference cannot be excluded.

There are two primary types of antithrombin deficiency: type I and type II. Type I antithrombin deficiency is characterized by an inadequate amount of normal antithrombin present. In this case, there is simply not enough antithrombin present to inactivate the coagulation factors. In type II antithrombin deficiency, the amount of antithrombin present is normal, but it does not function properly and is thus unable to carry out its normal functions. In many cases, the antithrombin in type I deficiencies has a problem binding to heparin, although there have been multiple other changes to the antithrombin molecule described. None of these conditions affect chromogenic assays, but there is a rare type II variant that might not be detected by chromogenic assays but is detected by clot-based assays. More recently, another rare variant, Asn2Ile, has been identified that is missed by chromogenic assays, and it is also missed by some clot-based assays[26]. Testing protein C while on warfarin therapy is not recommended because warfarin decreases protein C (and protein S) levels. However, if testing is inadvertently sent while on warfarin, the result with a chromogenic assay is typically higher than with clot-based assays.

2.3. Protein S

Protein S is an important anticoagulant protein, which acts as a non-enzymatic co-factor of activated protein C (APC) during inactivation of factor Va and VIIIa. Laboratory screening of protein S deficiency is complicated by the fact that protein S circulates in bloodstream in two forms, i.e. bound and free[27]. Forty percent of total protein S is represented by free protein S, which acts as the APC co-factor.

Protein S deficiency may be divided into three basic forms. Type I is characterized by a decrease in total protein S most often due to decreased synthesis, type II is characterized by decreased protein S activity and type III by a decreased level of free protein S and normal activity of total protein S.

Most deficits are type I or a combination of types I and III. At present very few cases of type II protein S deficiency have been described. The prevalence of protein S deficiency represents 1-2% of patients with deep venous thrombosis and 6% of families with thrombophilia. From a genetic viewpoint, 70 different mutations in the gene for protein S have been described to date.

The detection of protein S deficiency is complicated, because protein S circulated in the blood stream in two forms, i.e. bound protein S associated with C4b binding protein (60%) and free protein S (40%). The thrombotic risk potential constitutes only free protein S. Protein S activity may be determined using clot-based (aPTT, PT, Xa or RVV) assays. A number of factors may interfere with clot based assays. Lupus anticoagulants or direct thrombin inhibitors[28] can cause falsely elevated results. Factor V Leiden can cause falsely low results with PT-, Xa-, RVV-, and some aPTT-based assays[29]-[31]. With aPTT-based assays, elevated factor VIII can cause falsely low results because factor VIII shortens the aPTT in the assay.

Protein S free or total antigen assays do not suffer from similar limitations. Acute phase reactions (e.g., illness, inflammation) can falsely decrease protein S in vivo, and it is a common cause of low protein S activity or decreased free antigen results (but not total protein S antigen). This effect is attributed to C4b-binding protein, which becomes elevated during acute phase reactions. C4b-binding protein binds to protein S, thus reducing the amount of free protein S. When protein S is bound to C4b-binding protein, it is essentially inactive. The main disadvantage of free or total protein S antigen assays is that type II deficiencies will not be detected[32], but the majority of hereditary protein S deficiencies are type I (quantitative).

3. Factor V Leiden and APC resistance

The detection of Factor V Leiden (FVL) is usually performed as genetic confirmation of activated protein C (APC) resistance positivity. The classical assay for activated protein C resistance detects a ratio between a baseline activated partial thromboplastin time (aPTT) and the aPTT with APC. A variety of conditions can cause "falsely elevated" or "falsely decreased" ratios and interfere with this test, rendering it somewhat insensitive and nonspecific for diagnosing FVL, However, a positive result of APC resistance, due to acquired factors, may pose the same risk as the presence of the FVL mutation [33].

Elevated factor VIII (FVIII), the presence of a lupus anticoagulant, and certain drugs including oral contraceptives, estrogen, vitamin K antagonists, heparin, or direct thrombin inhibitors may interfere with the traditional aPTT-based APC assay. Improved assays are available, including the second-generation assay for activated protein C resistance, with sensitivity and specificity approaching 100% for the diagnosis of factor V Leiden[34]. The modification involves diluting the patient plasma into factor V-deficient plasma, thus minimizing the effect of factor V deficiencies and factor FVIII elevations that alter the baseline aPTT. Despite these changes, lupus anticoagulants may cause falsely low ratio results and direct thrombin inhibitors can cause falsely normal ratio results[35],[66].

Newer test options include Russell viper venom (RVV)-based assays, which uses the factor X activator from RVV. The reagent contains phospholipid designed to reduce lupus anticoagulant interference.

A factor Xa-based clotting assay is a third type of new assay for APC resistance. The method includes dilution into a proprietary reagent containing purified factors II, fibrinogen, protein S, and activated protein C. The inclusion of these factors presumably eliminates interference due to deficiencies or increased levels of these proteins.

While APC resistence positivity caused by presence of lupus anticoagulants is often considered to be „falsely elevated", several studies report that this parameter has some clinical significance.

While APC resistance positivity caused by lupus anticoagulants is often thought of as an "falsely elevated", some studies report that it have clinical significance.

Factor V Leiden can be detected by several DNA assays. In recent years, different molecular approaches, including restriction fragment length polymorphism (RFLP) and real-time PCR, have been developed to genotype single nucleotide polymorphisms (SNPs). Compared with more traditional methods such as RFLP, real-time PCR is a fast, simple, and accurate procedure for SNP genotyping of medium to large collections of samples. Real-time PCR analysis can be performed using various strategies[5]. In the hydrolysis assay, the probe and fluorescent chromogen is released by hydrolysis during PCR amplification and the free probe quantity is proportional to the fluorescence[37]. Fluorescence resonance energy transfer (FRET) is a method that distinguishes alleles by melting the products and monitoring the loss of fluorescence using an allele-specific oligonucleotide probe which hybridizes to specific sequences[38]-[40].

High-resolution melting analysis with LCGreen™ I is a newly designed analysis that detects heteroduplexes during homogeneous melting curve analysis with a new fluorescent DNA dye[41]. Genotyping of single-nucleotide polymorphisms (SNPs)1 by high-resolution melting analysis in products as large as 544 bp has been reported. This allows closed-tube, homogeneous allele-specific PCR genotyping [45],[46], on real-time PCR instruments without fluorescently labeled probes[42]-[44]. Heterozygotes are identified by a change in melting curve shape, and different homozygotes are distinguished by a change in melting temperature (Tm). However, it is still not clear whether all SNPs can be genotyped by this method[45]-[47].

Among the Caucasian population, factor V Leiden (factor V 1691G-A) is the most common genetic defect causing thrombosis[48]-[54]with a frequency between 2 and 15 % [49].. Factor V mutation was first described by Bertina et al in 1994 at the University of Leiden[55], based on the discovery of resistance to activated protein C (APC), which was first described in 1993[56]. The heterozygous form of factor V Leiden increases the risk of thrombosis 3 – 8x [49],[57],[58], while the homozygous form presents a risk which may be up to 80 times greater[59].

Factor V Leiden is present in up to 20% of patients with venous thrombosis[50],[57] and in over half of probands in selected families with thrombophilia making it the most common genetic abnormality in patients with thrombosis.

4. Pathophysiology of action FV Leiden mutation

FV plays a key role in both the procoagulation and anticoagulation cascade processes. In the activated form, it acts as a co-factor for FXa in the prothrombinase complex and as such catalyses the conversion of prothrombin to thrombin. In the inactive form FV acts as an APC co-factor in the regulatory activity of FVIIIa. In inherited and acquired defects, this double role allows FV to influence the manifestation of these disorders into hemorrhagic or thrombotic forms [60],[61]. To determine this manifestation, it is necessary to recognize precisely the procoagulation and anticoagulation forms of FV[63].

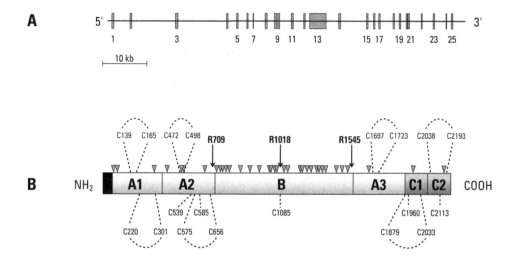

Figure 2. Schematic representation of the structure of FV

Unlike FV, FVa increases the FXa activated conversion of prothrombin in the prothrombinase complex. It may be expected that the cleaved B-domain allosterically inhibits the binding of FV in the active site of FXa [63].

The mechanism by which FVa acts on FXa is not completely understood. Based on the latest works, it may be assumed that FVa increases the binding affinity of FXa to phospholipids by about 100x. In addition, it was determined that FVa in the prothrombinase complex does not change the binding site of FXa, but instead increases the affinity of the prothrombinase complex to prothrombin and ensures an increase in binding sites.

The co-factor activity of FVa is balanced by APC, which proteolytically cleaves FVa at the Arg306, Arg506 and Arg679 sites of the heavy chain. The weakest inactivation is seen during cleavage at the Arg679 site. Latest discoveries suggest two pathophysiological models of FVa cleavage. The first model assumes preferential cleavage at the Arg506 site followed by cleavage at the Arg306 site. Alternatively, FVa may be inactivated directly by cleavage at the Arg306 site. Cleavage at the Arg506 site also decreases the affinity of FVa to FXa, while cleavage at the Arg306 site causes complete inactivation of FVa [64].

5. Anticoagulation function of FVa

Aside from its procoagulation function, FVa also possesses an anticoagulation function, which is expressed as APC activation. In this case it is a cofactor in the proteolytic cleavage of FVIIIa[65]. Recent experimental works supports this model where the addition of purified FV renewed the function of APC in both healthy patients and in families with the Leiden mutation. The experiments utilized measured generation of thrombin.

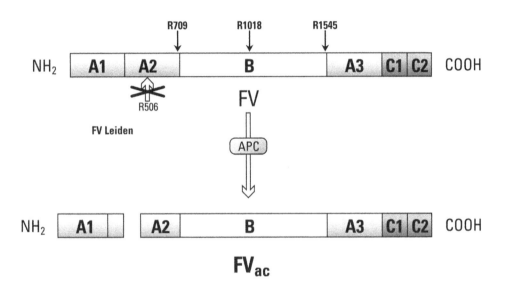

Figure 3. Anticoagulation structure of FV[59]

Thus if the anticoagulation function of FV is required, cleavage must occur in position Arg506. Unlike APC mediated cleavage in sites Arg306 and Arg679, which does not exhibit anticoagulation activity.

6. FV and thrombophilia

Such described pathways of FV activation point to the balance of pro- and anticoagulation activity of factor V and its significance in maintaining haemostatic equilibrium. The pathways of FV activation describe the mututal balance of both pro- and anticoagulation activity of factor V and its significance in maintaining haemostatic equilibrium.

APC resistance is an in vitro described phenomenon, which is characterized by a slight anticoagulation response to APC in plasma. Such decreased sensitivity to APC leads to inadequate regulation of thrombin production. As such, APC resistance is associated with an increased risk of developing thrombosis. APC resistance is associated with FV Leiden mutation in up to 90 % of cases.

FV Leiden mutation significantly influences the pro- and anticoagulation balance of FVa. The Leiden mutation, which leads to the disappearance of the Arg506 cleavage site, causes an insufficient decrease of the procoagulation activity of FVa, which explains the presence of procoagulation states in carriers of the Leiden mutation.

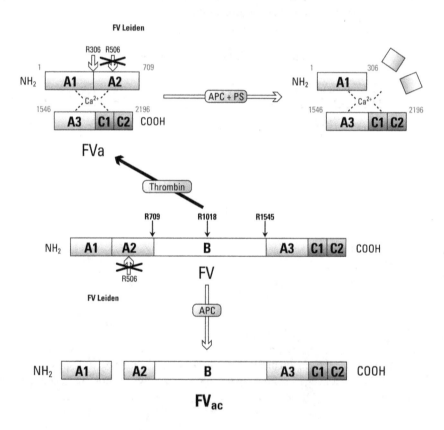

Figure 4. A schematic illustration of the activation of FV to procoagulation and anticoagulation forms

The discovery of a second pathway of action of FVa, where via APC it acts as a co-factor during proteolytic cleavage of FVIIIa aids us in establishing the effect of the Leiden mutation. Since FV with the Leiden mutation does not contain a cleavage site in the position Arg506, the anticoagulation form FVac cannot be produced and therefore there is only weak co-factor activity of APC during FVIII proteolysis.

7. Prothrombin 20210A

Mutations in the 3′- untranslated region of the prothrombin gene in the position 20210 G-A are associated with an increased level of prothrombin and as such present an increased risk of developing thrombosis[66]. This mutation was described with a high prevalence (up to 18%) in families with thrombosis and in 6.2% of patients with first thrombosis[66].

F II 20210G-A mutation in the gene for prothrombin was found through linkage analysis in families with a history of venous thrombosis and no other congenital or acquired thrombophilic risk factors[67]. The mutation is located in the 3 'gene region, which already does not overwrite to the protein. The mutation is located in the 3 'gene region, which already does not overwrite to the protein. Therefore, it appears difficult to develop a specific functional coagulation tests based FII activity determination. However, in large clinical studies found significantly elevated levels of prothrombin mutations in patients with FII 20210 GThere is no evidence that the homozygous mutation carriers have a higher level of prothrombin than heterozygous. The pathophysiologic influence of the mutation is not yet fully explained. The original view was that the mutation alters the conformation of the pre-mRNA 3'UTR, which has an increased affinity for the production of polyA end. This causes an increased concentration of mRNA with an increase in protein synthesis, so the greater the level of prothrombin in plasma[68]. Later work demonstrated that the mutation does not affect the mRNA level, but instead 3' cleavage/polyadenylation, which affects abnormal properties of mRNAs[69]. Finally, recent work showing abnormal properties mRNA 20210A mutation in the 3'UTR, which cause the emergence of polyA preferentially in the presence of this mutation in the mRNA[70].

The prevalence of this mutation in the normal population is 1.7% in northern Europe and 3% in southern Europe[71],[72]. This mutation is very rare among people of African and Asian origin. It was found that originated as a founder effect until after the separation of Caucasian populations [73]-[76].

Apart from this, the mutation may represent an additional risk factor for spontaneous abortions especially during the first trimester[77]. The risk of venous thrombosis is significantly increased in women with prothrombin mutation during pregnancy and after childbirth,and the frequency of thrombosis further increases in the presence of an additional risk factor, which - among others - can be factor V Leiden[78]. Prothrombin mutation may also affect the risk of arterial thrombosis, but this has not been clearly demonstrated yet. In a large group of 3028 patients, a statistically significant relationship between the mentioned mutations and ischemic stroke (odds ratio 1.44) [79] was demonstrated. Ingeneral the risk of spontaneous recurrent thromboembolic events is the same in patients with mutations without such mutations[80].

8. Potential genetic thrombophilic states

8.1. Plasminogen activator inhibitor-1 mutation

The plasminogen activator inhibitor-1 (PAI-1) mutation is a single base insertion or deletion at position -675 (4G/5G) in the promoter region of the PAI-1 gene, which is associated with

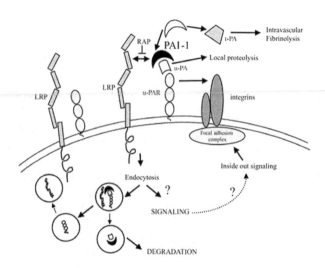

Figure 5. Schematic action PAI-1 in regulation mechanism of fibrinolytic system

higher levels of PAI-1 transcripts and also higher plasma activity of PAI-1[81]. In the PAI-1 -
675 4G/5G mutation, the 4G site binds an enhancer element only, whereas the 5G allele binds
both enhancer and suppressor elements. As a result individuals with 4G/5G or 4G/4G genotypes have an increased level of transcription and consequently a higher PAI-1 protein level
than individuals with 5G/5G polymorphism. Because PAI-1 is a rapid inhibitor of tissue
plasminogen activator (t-PA), the 4G/5G variant of mutation can increase the activity of PAI-1
and decrease the conversion of plasminogen to plasmin, which causes decreased fibrin
degeneration and increased clot stabilization.

Under physiological conditions, PAI-1 is released into the circulation and the extracellular
space by only a few cells: liver cells, smooth muscle cells (SMC), adipocytes, and platelets are
the major sources of PAI-1. This results in plasma levels of only 5–20 ng/ml of active PAI-1,
sufficient to control fibrinolysis and extracellular proteolysis.

Under pathological conditions, however, several other tissues secrete quite large amounts of
PAI-1: tumor cells, endothelial cells in response to inflammatory cytokines, and other inflam-
mation-activated cells. High PAI-1 plasma levels are consistently found in patients with severe
sepsis but also with other acute or chronic inflammatory diseases such as atherosclerosis. PAI-1
is upregulated by inflammatory cytokines and may therefore be regarded as a marker for an
ongoing inflammatory process. It is of major importance, however, that no classic inflammatory response element was found in the PAI-1 promoter region, and it is still unclear how PAI-1
expression is upregulated during inflammation[82].

8.2. Fibrinogen

Fibrinogen is a 340-kDa glycoprotein produced in the liver with a plasma concentration of 180
- 450 mg/dl. It consists of two monomers linked by a disulfide bond. Each monomer consists

of three polypeptide chains encoded by three distinct genes: Aa, Bb and γ. It binds to the platelet through the glycoprotein IIb/IIIa receptor and, therefore, is highly involved in the thrombotic processes. It also has a direct effect on the vascular wall and blood viscosity. An association between increased circulating levels of fibrinogen and the development of arterial thrombosis has been demonstrated[83],[84]. The mechanisms that explain the association between increased fibrinogen and AMI include increased fibrin formation, increased blood viscosity, platelet hyperaggregability and an increased proliferation of vascular endothelial and smooth muscle cells[85]. In addition, fibrinogen is an acute phase reactant and possibly an indicator of chronic inflammation associated with atherosclerosis.

There are several polymorphisms identified in the genes that code the three polypeptide chains and are associated with increased concentration of circulating fibrinogen (>500 mg/dl). From the functional point of view, the most relevant are those in the β chain: Arg448Lis, -148 C/T, -455 G/A and 854 G/A, with the last two having the most pathophysiological interest due to their association with the development of vascular disease. The genotype -455A is present in 10-20% of the general population and is correlated with an increase of 10% high concentration of fibrinogen, prevalence of other mutations not specifically described in current literature. Some studies[86] showed an association between the -455 polymorphism and an increased risk for arterial thrombosis.

9. Coagulation factor VII (FVII)

Factor VII is a single polypeptide chain, 406-amino acid glycoprotein with a weight of ~50,000 Da. It is vitamin K dependent protein, synthesized in the liver and has a plasma concentration of 500 ng/mL. FVII is transformed into its activated form (FVIIa) by binding with tissue factor (TF). The TF:FVIIa complex converts Factor IX and Factor X to their active forms, FIXa and FXa. Recent studies have described an association between an increased plasma concentration of FVII and development of arterial thrombosis[87]

In contrast, polymorphism Arg (R) 353Gln (Q) in the FVII gene is associated with a 20-25% decreased plasma concentration of FVII.[88]

In addition, several studies[89],[90] have demonstrated that plasma concentration of FVII is lower in subjects homozygous for the 353Gln allele compared with those homozygous for the 353Arg allele.

In contrast, other studies have been unable to corroborate the association of the polymorphism R/Q353 with AMI or increase in plasma concentration of FVII in subjects with Arg/Arg genotype[91].

10. Polymorphisms in platelets

Platelets play an important role in the development of acute coronary syndromes. Platelets possess glycoprotein receptors on the surface membrane which participate in platelet activation, degranulation and aggregation. These receptors belong to the family of integrins (aIIb β3) and are highly polymorphic, which often produces an antigenic alteration of the glycoprotein. The most frequent polymorphisms present in these glycoproteins are receptors for von Willebrand factor (vWF) (GPIb-IX, GIIb-III), a in the protein receptor for collagen (GPIa-IIa), and in the receptor for fibrinogen (GPIIb-IIIa).

The most abundant glycoprotein on the platelet membrane is the GPIIb-IIIa complex. Inactivated platelets bind through GIIb-IIIa complex to vWF and to fibrinogen. This polymorphism consists of a thymine substitution for cytosine in the 1565 position in exon 2 of the GPIII gene[92]. Approximately 25% of the population of northern Europe is a carrier of at least one allele PLA2 (PLA1/A2). Several studies described an association between this polymorphism and AMI in patients <60 years[93], ACS[94] and atherothrombosis[95]. Many studies have attempted to establish an association between the presence of allele PLA2 and coronary artery disease, but results are still contradictory.

11. Hyperhomocysteinemia

Increased levels of homocysteine are associated with an increased risk of thrombosis[96]-[98]. Two studies performed on an undivided group of patients showed that a level above 18.5 μmol/l in 5 % (10 % respectively) of tested subjects led to a two-fold increase in the risk of thrombotic episodes[99]-[101]. This means that hyperhomocysteinemia represents 5 – 10 % of all thrombotic episodes.

Hyperhomocysteinemia may develop due to genetic or acquired dispositions[99]. Acquired dispositions primarily include low vitamin intake or resorption (B6, B12, folic acid), which leads to an increase in homocysteine level[101],[102]. Genetic factors include the very rare cystathione β-synthase deficit, whose homozygous form represents classical hyperhomocysteinemia with very high levels[103], and on the other hand the very common variant of the methyltetrahydrofolate reductase (MTHFR) gene, which leads to the thermolabile enzyme variant with a slightly increased homocysteine level[104]-[106]. Currently, direct association between the MTHFR 677TT variant, increased homocysteine level and risk of developing thrombosis is not distinctly established[107].

12. Conclusion

The elucidation of the precise pathogenesis of action leads to the conclusion that to explain the clinical expression of thrombophilic conditions, it is most important to understand the interaction of at least one genetically dependent thrombophilia with one or more acquired conditions.

Determination of thrombophilic markers is necessary to evaluate the risk of thrombophilia in the examined patients. The degree of risk depends largely on the choice of methods for testing individual markers and their specificity. Another important reality in the interpretation of tests are interfering factors for each test.

Uncritical interpretation of laboratory results can lead to misdiagnosis and thrombophilia testing exemplifies this. If possible errors and overdiagnosis are to be avoided, the following points should be respected: Normal ranges for antithrombin and proteins C or S levels are wide and patients with deficiency may have levels that are only slightly below normal. Repeated testing is often required for diagnostic accuracy. For example, laboratory quality assurance data have shown that for protein S in particular the rate of laboratory error in diagnosis can be as high as 20%. Pregnancy induces a state of resistance to the anticoagulant effect of activated protein C, which mimics the presence of factor V Leiden. Pregnancy and OCP use lead to a fall in plasma protein S concentration. Antithrombin concentration is reduced in acute thrombosis, by heparin treatment and in pre-eclampsia state. Proteins C and S are vitamin K dependent and their concentrations are reduced by warfarin treatment. Even if the above potential pitfalls are avoided, there is no indication to routine testing for heritable thrombophilia at presentation with acute VTE, as clinical management is not influenced by the results.

Concerning the determination of mutation FII 20210 G / A, the situation is quite the opposite. Screening test shows high interference with the current status, therefore it is completely unusable and direct molecular genetic analysis of point mutations FII 20210 G-A.

The identification of potential genetic causes of thrombophilia, such as mutation of fibrinogen, platelet receptor, PAI-1, F VII and homocysteine are designed for testing the rare causes of thrombophilia in thrombotic centers. Howeever, they can be beneficial to clarify complex cases of thrombophilia especially if associated with repeated manifestations in the family.

Genetic testing is a separate part of the diagnosis of thrombophilia. Generally, it is not intended for screening the universal population, but only to determine the causes of thrombophilia in defined groups of patients - young patients with a positive family history of thrombophilia, in patients with previous thrombosis under 45 years of age, patients with the manifestation of thrombosis in an unusual site (e.g. portal vein), and at women in pregnancy or with using oral contraceptives.

Author details

Ludek Slavik*

Address all correspondence to: ludek.slavik@fnol.cz

Hemato-oncology Clinic, Faculty of Medicine and Dentistry Palacky University Olomouc, Czech Republic

References

[1] Picard V, Prescot I, Scarabin PY, et al. Antithrombin Cambridge II (A384S): Prevalence in patients of the Paris Thrombosis Study (PATHROS). Blood 2007; 110: 2777–2778.

[2] Vorlova Z., Hrachovinova I., Matyskova M. Probability of thrombosis in patients with factor V Leiden. Thromb.Haemost. 1997; 78/1:309.

[3] Chrobák, L., Dulíček, P.: Resistance to activated protein C as pathogenic factor of venous thromboembolism. - Acta Medica (Hradec Králové). - 1996; 39,(2):55-62.

[4] Martinelli I, Mannucci PM, De Stefano V, et al. Different sisks of thrombosis in four coagulation defects associated with inherited thrombophilia: a study of 150 families. Blood 1998; 92: 2353-2358

[5] Hluší, A., Slavík, L., Úlehlová, J., Krčová, V., Indrák, K. Global assessment of haemostagic function - Part I. Thrombin generation test Transfuze a Hematologie Dnes 2010;16 (2), pp. 65-70

[6] Egeberg O. Inherited antithrombin deficiency causing thrombophilia. Thromb Diath Haemorrh. 1965; 13:516-530.

[7] Thaler E, Lechner K. Antithrombin III deficiency and thromboembolism. Clin Haematol. 1981; 10:369-390.

[8] Demers C, Ginsberg JS, Hirsh J, Henderson P, Blajchman MA. Thrombosis in antithrombin III deficient persons: report of a large kindred and literature review. Ann Intern Med. 1992; 116:754-761.

[9] Hirsh J, Piovella F, Pini M. Congenital antithrombin III deficiency: incidence and clinical features. Am J Med. 1989; 87:34-38.

[10] Lane DA, Mannucci PM, Bauer KA, Bertina RM, Bochkov NP, Boulyjenkov V et al. Inherited Thrombophilia: Part 1. Thromb Haemost. 1996; 76:651-662.

[11] Khor B,Van Cott EM. Laboratory tests for antithrombin deficiency. Am J Hematol 2010; 85: 947–950.

[12] Ungerstedt JS,Schulman S,Egberg N, et al. Discrepancy between antithrombin activity methods revealed in Antithrombin Stockholm: Do factor Xa-based methods overestimate antithrombin activity in some patients? Blood 2002; 99: 2271–2272.

[13] Lindahl TL,Baghaei F,Blixter IF, et al. Effects of the oral, direct thrombin inhibitor dabigatran on five common coagulation assays. Thromb Haemost 2011; 105: 371–378.

[14] Rossi E,Chiusolo P,Za T, et al. Report of a novel kindred with antithrombin heparin-binding site variant (47 Arg to His): Demand for an automated progressive antithrombin assay to detect molecular variants with low thrombotic risk. Thromb Haemost 2007; 98: 695–697.

[15] Tait RC,Walker ID,Perry DJ, et al. Prevalence of antithrombin deficiency in the healthy population. Br J Haematol 1994; 87: 106–112.

[16] Corral J,Hernandez-Espinosa D,Soria JM, et al. Antithrombin Cambridge II (A384S): An underestimated genetic risk factor for venous thrombosis. Blood 2007; 109: 4258–4263.

[17] Griffin JH, Evatt B, Zimmerman TS, Kleiss AJ, Wideman C. Deficiency of protein C in congenital thrombotic disease. J Clin Invest. 1981; 68:1370-1373.

[18] Allaart CF, Poort SR, Rosendaal FR, Reitsma PH, Bertina RM, Briët E. Increased risk of venous thrombosis in carriers of protein C deficiency defect. Lancet. 1993; 341:134-138.

[19] Broekmans AW, Veltkamp JJ, Bertina RM. Congenital protein C deficiency and venous thromboembolism: a study of three Dutch families. N Engl J Med. 1983; 309:340-344.

[20] Allaart CF, Poort SR, Rosendaal FR, Reitsma PH, Bertina RM, Briët E. Increased risk of venous thrombosis in carriers of protein C deficiency defect. Lancet. 1993; 341:134-138.

[21] Koeleman BPC, Reitsma PH, Allaart CF, Bertina RM. APC-resistance as an additional risk factor for thrombosis in protein C deficient families. Blood. 1994; 84:1031-1035.

[22] Heijboer H, Brandjes DPM, Büller HR, Sturk A, Ten Cate JW. Deficiencies of coagulation-inhibiting and fibrinolytic proteins in outpatients with deep-vein thrombosis. N Engl J Med. 1990; 323:1512-1516.

[23] Mateo J, Oliver A, Borrell M, Sala N, Fontcuberta J, the EMET Group. Laboratory evaluation and clinical characteristics of 2,132 consecutive unselected patients with venous thromboembolism-results of the Spanish multicentric study on thrombophilia(EMET-study). Thromb Haemost. 1997; 77: 444-451.

[24] Cooper PC,Cooper SM,Goodfellow KJ, et al. Evaluation of a new venom-based clotting assay of protein C. Int J Lab Hematol 2008; 30: 437–443.

[25] Cooper PC,Siddiq S,Morse C, et al. Marked discrepancy between coagulometric protein C activity assays with the pro-thrombotic protein C Asn2Ile substitution. Int J Lab Hematol 2011; 33: 451–456.

[26] Walker I.D. et al. Guidelines on the Investigation and Management of Thrombophilia. J. Clin Path, 43, 1990, 703 – 709.

[27] Walenga JM,Drenth AF,Mayuga M, et al. Transition from argatroban to oral anticoagulation with phenprocoumon or acenocoumarol: Effect on coagulation factor testing. Clin Appl Thromb Hemost 2008; 14: 325–331.

[28] D'Angelo SV,Mazzola G,Della Valle P, et al. Variable interference of activated protein C resistance in the measurement of protein S activity by commercial assays. Thromb Res 1995; 77: 375.

[29] Faioni EM,Boyer-Neumann C,Franchi F, et al. Another protein S functional assay is sensitive to resistance to activated protein C. Thromb Haemost 1994; 72: 648.

[30] Jennings I,Kitchen S,Cooper P, et al. Sensitivity of functional protein S assays to protein S deficiency: A comparative study of three commercial kits. J Thromb Haemost 2003; 1: 1112.

[31] Khor B,Van Cott EM. Laboratory evaluation of hypercoagulability. Clin Lab Med 2009; 29: 339–366.

[32] Marlar RA,Gausman JN. Protein S Abnormalities: A diagnostic nightmare. Am J Hematol 2011; 86: 418–421.

[33] Rodeghiero F, Tosetto A. Activated protein C resistance and factor V Leiden mutation are independent risk factors for venous thromboembolism. Ann Intern Med 1999; 130: 643–50.

[34] Gibson NJ (2007) The use of real-time PCR methods in DNA sequence variation analysis. Mol Cell Probes 363:171–176

[35] Sevall JS (2001) Rapid allelic discrimination from real-time DNA amplification. Methods 25:452–455

[36] Didenko VV (2001) DNA probes using fluorescence resonance energy transfer (FRET): designs and applications. Biotechniques 31(5):1106–1121

[37] Holland PM, Abramson RD, Watson R, Gelfand DH (2001) Detection of specific polymerase chain reaction product by utilizing the 5′–3′ exonuclease activity of Thermus aquaticus DNA polymerase. Biochemistry 88:7276–7280

[38] Lay MJ, Wittwer CT (1997) Real-time fluorescence genotyping of factor V Leiden during rapid-cycle PCR. ClinChem 43(12):2262–2267

[39] Liew M, Pryor R, Palais R, Meadows C, Erali M, Lyon E, Wittwer C (2004) Genotyping of single-nucleotide polymorphisms by high-resolution melting of small amplicons. Clin Chem 50(7):1156–1164

[40] Parks SB, Popovich BW, Press RD (2001) Real-time polymerase chain reaction with fluorescent hybridization probes for the detection of prevalent mutations causing common thrombophilic and iron overload phenotypes. Am J Clin Pathol 115:439–447

[41] Wittwer CT, Reed GH, Gundry CN, Vandersteen JG, Pryor RJ. High-resolution genotyping by amplicon melting analysis using LCGreen. Clin Chem 2003;49:853–60.

[42] Lay MJ, Wittwer CT. Real-time fluorescence genotyping of factor V Leiden during rapid-cycle PCR. Clin Chem 1997;43:2262-2267.

[43] Livak KJ, Flood SJ, Marmaro J, Giusti W, Deetz K. Oligonucleotides with fluorescent dyes at opposite ends provide a quenched probe system useful for detecting PCR product and nucleic acid hybridization. PCR Methods Appl 1995;4:357-362.

[44] Crockett AO, Wittwer CT. Fluorescein-labeled oligonucleotides for real-time pcr: using the inherent quenching of deoxyguanosine nucleotides. Anal Biochem 2001;290:89-97.

[45] Angelini A, Di Febbo C, Baccante G, Di Nisio M, Di Ilio C, Cuccurullo F, Porreca E. Identification of three genetic risk factors for venous thrombosis using a multiplex allele-specific PCR assay: comparison of conventional and new alternative methods for the preparation of DNA from clinical samples. J Thromb Thrombolysis. 2003 Dec;16(3): 189-93.

[46] Ugozzoli LA, Hamby K. Four-color multiplex 5′ nuclease assay for the simultaneous detection of the factor V Leiden and the prothrombin G20210A mutations. Mol Cell Probes. 2004 Jun;18(3):161-6.

[47] Bianchi M, Emanuele E, Davin A, Gagliardi S, Cova E, Meli V, Trotti R, Cereda C. Comparison of three methods for genotyping of prothrombotic polymorphisms. Clin Exp Med. 2010 Dec;10(4):269-72. Epub 2010 Apr 29.

[48] Reitsma PH, Rosendaal FR. Past and future of genetic research in thrombosis. J Thromb Haemost. 2007, Jul 5; Suppl 1:264-9.

[49] Rees DC, Cox M, Clegg JB. World distribution of factor V Leiden. Lancet. 1995; 346:1133-1134.

[50] Rosendaal FR, Koster T, Vandenbroucke JP, Reitsma PH. High risk of thrombosis in patients homozygous for factor V Leiden (activated protein C resistance). Blood. 1995; 85:1504-1508.23.

[51] Ridker PM, Miletich JP, Hennekens CH, Buring JE. Ethnic distribution of factor V Leiden in 4047 men and women. JAMA. 1997; 277, 1305-1307.

[52] Vorlova Z., Hrachovinova I., Matyskova M. Probability of thrombosis in patients with factor V Leiden. Thromb.Haemost. 1997; 78/1:309.

[53] Chrobák, L., Dulíček, P.: Resistance to activated protein C as pathogenic factor of venous thromboembolism. - Acta Medica (Hradec Králové). - 1996; 39,(2):55-62.

[54] Dulíček P., Šafářová M., Chrobák L. Mutace FV Leiden – nejčastější rizikový faktor pro vznik žilní trombózy. Hematológia a transfuziológia. 1997; 4:6-9.

[55] Bertina RM, Koeleman RPC, Koster T, Rosendaal FR, Dirven RJ, De Ronde H et al. Mutation in blood coagulation factor V associated with resistance to activated protein C. Nature. 1994; 369:64-67.

[56] Dahlbäck B, Carlsson M, Svensson PJ. Familial thrombophilia due to a previously unrecognised mechanism characterized by poor anticoagulant response to activated protein C: prediction of a cofactor to activated protein C. Proc Natl Acad Sci USA. 1993; 90:1004-1008.

[57] Koster T, Rosendaal FR, De Ronde H, Briët E, Vandenbroucke JP, Bertina RM. Venous thrombosis due to a poor anticoagulant response to activated protein C: Leiden Thrombophilia Study. Lancet. 1993; 342:1503-1506.

[58] Ridker PM, Hennekens CH, Lindpainter K, Stampfer MJ, Eisenberg PR, Miletich JP. Mutation in the gene coding for coagulation factor V and the risk of myocardial infarction, stroke, and venous thrombosis in apparently healthy men. N Engl J Med. 1995; 332:912-917.

[59] Anderson FA, Wheeler HB, Goldberg RJ, Hosmer DW, Patwardhan NA, Jovanovic B et al. A population based perspective of the hospital incidence and case-fatality rates of deep vein thrombosis and pulmonary embolism. The Worcester DVT study. Arch Intern Med. 1991; 151:933-938.

[60] Cripe LD, Moore KD, Kane WH. Structure of the gene for human coagulation factor V. Biochemistry 1992; 31: 3777–3785.

[61] Jenny RJ, Pittman DD, Toole JJ, et al. Complete cDNA and derived amino acid sequence of human factor V. Proc Natl Acad Sci USA 1987; 84: 4846–4850.

[62] Segers K., Dahlbäck B, Nicolaes G. Coagulation factor V and thrombophilia: Background and mechanisms. Thromb Haemost. 2007 Sep; 98(3):530-42.

[63] Husten EJ, Esmon CT, Johnson AE. The active site of blood coagulation factor Xa. Its distance from the phospholipid surface and its conformational sensitivity to components of the prothrombinase complex. J Biol Chem 1987; 262: 12953–12961.

[64] Yegneswaran S, Fernandez JA, Griffin JH. Factor Va increases the affinity of factor Xa for prothrombin: a binding study using a novel photoactivable thiol-specific fluorescent probe. Chem Biol 2002; 9: 485–494.

[65] Dahlbäck B, Carlsson M, Svensson PJ. Familial thrombophilia due to a previously unrecognized mechanism characterized by poor anticoagulant response to activated protein C: prediction of a cofactor to activated protein C. Proc Natl Acad Sci USA 1993; 90:1004–1008.

[66] Poort SR, Rosendaal FR, Reitsma PH, Bertina RM. A common genetic variation in the 3′-untranslated region of the prothrombin gene is associated with elevated plasma prothrombin levels and an increase in venous thrombosis. Blood. 1996; 88:3698-3703.

[67] Poort, S. R.; Rosendaal, F. R.; Reitsma, P. H.; Bertina, R. M. : A common genetic variation in the 3-prime-untranslated region of the prothrombin gene is associated with elevated plasma prothrombin levels and an increase in venous thrombosis. Blood 88: 3698-3703, 1996.

[68] Gehring, N. H.; Frede, U.; Neu-Yilik, G.; Hundsdoerfer, P.; Vetter, B.; Hentze, M. W.; Kulozik, A. E. : Increased efficiency of mRNA 3-prime end formation: a new genetic mechanism contributing to hereditary thrombophilia. Nature Genet. 28: 389-392, 2001.

[69] Eleanor S. Pollak, Ho-Sun Lam, and J. Eric Russell The G20210A mutation does not affect the stability of prothrombin mRNA in vivo. Blood 2002 ;100(1):359-62.

[70] Ceelie H, Spaargaren-van Riel CC, Bertina RM, Vos HL. G20210A is a functional mutation in the prothrombin gene; effect on protein levels and 3′-end formation. J Thromb Haemost. 2: 119-27. 2004

[71] Rosendaal, F. R.; Doggen, C. J. M.; Zivelin, A.; Arruda, V. R.; Aiach, M.; Siscovick, D. S.; Hillarp, A.; Watzke, H. H.; Bernardi, F.; Cumming, A. M.; Preston, F. E.; Reitsma, P. H. : Geographic distribution of the 20210 G to a prothrombin variant. Thromb. Haemost. 79: 706-708, 1998.

[72] Rosendaal FR, Doggen CJM, Zivelin A, Arruda VR, Aiach M, Siscovick DS et al. Geographic distribution of the 20210 G to A prothrombin variant. Thromb Haemost. 1998; 79:706-708.

[73] Zivelin, A.; Rosenberg, N.; Faier, S.; Kornbrot, N.; Peretz, H.; Mannhalter, C.; Horellou, M. H.; Seligsohn, U. : A single genetic origin for the common prothrombotic G20210A polymorphism in the prothrombin gene. Blood 92: 1119-1124, 1998.

[74] Rees, D. C.; Chapman, N. H.; Webster, M. T.; Guerreiro, J. F.; Rochette, J.; Clegg, J. B. : Born to clot: the European burden. Brit. J. Haemat. 105: 564-566, 1999.

[75] Matýšková M., Buliková A., Šlechtová M., Janků L. The prevalence of the prothrombin mutation 20210A in Brno, XV meeting of the ISH - African and European division, Final programme and abstracts, 124.

[76] Souto JC, Coll I, Llobet D, del Río E, Oliver A, Mateo J, Borrell M et al. The prothrombin 20210A allele is the most present genetic risk factor for venous thromboembolism in the Spanish population. Thromb Haemost. 1998; 80:366-369.

[77] Pihusch, R.; Buchholz, T.; Lohse, P.; Rubsamen, H.; Rogenhofer, N.; Hasbargen, U.; Hiller, E.; Thaler, C. J. : Thrombophilic gene mutations and recurrent spontaneous abortion: prothrombin mutation increases the risk in the first trimester. Am. J. Reprod. Immun. 2001, 46: 124-131.

[78] Samama MM, Rached RA, Horellou MH, Aquilanti S, Mathieux VG, Bureau G, Elalamy I, Conard J. Pregnancy-associated venous thromboembolism (VTE) in combined heterozygous factor V Leiden (FVL) and prothrombin (FII) 20210 A mutation and in heterozygous FII single gene mutation alone. British Journal of Haematology, 123, 327–334, 2003.

[79] Casas, J. P.; Hingorani, A. D.; Bautista, L. E.; Sharma, P. : Meta-analysis of genetic studies in ischemic stroke: thirty-two genes involving approximately 18000 cases and 58000 controls. Arch. Neurol. 61: 1652-1662, 2004.

[80] De Stefano, V.; Martinelli, I.; Mannucci, P. M.; Paciaroni, K.; Chiusolo, P.; Casorelli, I.;Rossi, E.; Leone, G. : The risk of recurrent deep venous thrombosis among heterozygous carriers of both factor V Leiden and the G20210A prothrombin mutation. New Eng. J. Med. 341: 801-806, 1999.

[81] Grubic N, Stegnar M, Peternel P, Kaider A, and Binder BR. A novel G/A and the 4G/5G polymorphism within the promoter of the plasminogen activator inhibitor-1 gene in patients with deep vein thrombosis. Thromb Res 84: 431 443, 1996.

[82] Binder BR, Christ G, Gruber F, Grubic N, Hufnagl P, Krebs M, Mihaly J, Prager GW. Plasminogen activator inhibitor 1: physiological and pathophysiological roles. News Physiol Sci. 2002 Apr;17:56-61.

[83] Meade TW, Mellows S, Brozovic M, Miller GJ, Chakrabarti RR, North WR, et al. Haemostatic function and ischaemic heart disease: principal results of the Northwick Park Heart Study. Lancet 1986;2:533-537.

[84] Heinrich J, Balleisen L, Schulte H, Assmann G, van de Loo J. Fibrinogen and factor VII in the prediction of coronary risk: results from the PROCAM study in healthy men. Arterioscler Thromb 1994;14:54-59.

[85] Folsom AR. Haemostatic risk factors for atherothrombotic disease: an epidemiologic view. Thromb Haemost 2001;86:366-373.

[86] Behague I, Poirier O, Nicaud V, Evans A, Arveiler D, Luc G, et al. Beta fibrinogen gene polymorphisms are associated with plasma fibrinogen and coronary artery disease in patients with myocardial infarction: The ECTIM Study. Etude Cas-temoins sur l'Infarctus du Myocarde. Circulation 1996;93:440-449.

[87] Carvalho de Sousa J, Bruckert E, Giral P, Soria C, Truffert J, Mirshami MC, de Gennes JL, Caen JP Plasma factor VII, triglyceride concentration and fibrin degradation products in primary hyperlipidemia:a clinical and laboratory study. Haemostasis, 1989; 19(2):83-90.

[88] Green F, Kelleher C, Wilkes H, Temple A, Meade T, Humphries S. A common genetic polymorphism associated with lower coagulation factor VII levels in healthy individuals. Arterioscler Thromb 1991;11:540-546.

[89] Iacoviello L, Di Castelnuovo A, De Knijff P, D'Orazio A, Amore C, Arboretti R, et al. Polymorphism in the coagulation factor VII gene and the risk of myocardial infarction. N Engl J Med 1998;338:79-85.

[90] Corral J, González-Conejero R, Lozano ML, Rivera J, Vicente V. Genetic polymorphisms of factor VII are not associated with arterial thrombosis. Blood Coagul Fibrinolysis 1998;9:267-272.

[91] Ekström M, Silveira A, Bennermo M, Eriksson P, Tornvall P. Coagulation factor VII and inflammatory markers in patients with coronary heart disease. Blood Coagul Fibrinolysis 2007;18:473-477.

[92] Newman PJ, Derbes RS, Aster RH. The human platelet alloantigens, PIA1 and PIA2, are associated with a leucine 33/proline33 amino acid polymorphism in membrane glycoprotein IIIa, and are distinguishable by DNA typing. J Clin Invest 1989;83:1778-1781.

[93] Weiss EJ, Bray PF, Tayback M, Schulman SP, Kickler TS, Becker Isordia-Salas et al. Volume 78, No. 1, January-February 2010 91

[94] Carter AM, Catto AJ, Bamford JM, Grant PJ. Platelet GP IIIa PIA and GP Ib variable number tandem repeat polymorphism and markers of platelet activation in acute stroke. Arterioscler Thromb Vasc Biol 1998;18:1124-1131.

[95] Mikkelsson J, Perola M, Laippala P, Savolainen V, Pajarinen J, Lalu K, et al. Glycoprotein IIIa PI (A) polymorphism associates with progression of coronary artery disease and with myocardial infarction in an autopsy series of middle-aged men who died suddenly. Arterioscler Thromb Vasc Biol 1999;19:2573-2578.

[96] Falcon CR, Cattaneo M, Panzeri D, Martinelli I, Mannucci PM. High prevalence of hyperhomocyst(e)inemia in patients with juvenile venous thrombosis. Arterioscler Thromb. 1994; 14:1080-1083.

[97] Den Heijer M, Koster T, Blom HJ, Bos GMJ, Briët E, Reitsma PH et al. Hyperhomocysteinemia as a risk factor for deep-vein thrombosis. N Engl J Med. 1996; 334:759-762.

[98] Simioni P, Prandoni P, Burlina A, Tormene D, Sardella C, Ferrari V et al. Hyperhomocysteinemia and deep-vein thrombosis: a case-control study. Thromb Haemost. 1996; 76:883-886.

[99] Hyánek J., Hoffman R. Hyperhomocysteinémie a její diagnostický význam u cévních onemocnění. Praktická flebologie. 1997; 2:61-71.

[100] D'Angelo A, Selhub J. Homocysteine and thrombotic disease. Blood. 1997; 90:1-11.

[101] Kang SS, Wong PWK, Norusis M. Homocysteinemia due to folate deficiency. Metabolism. 1987; 36:458-462.

[102] Kang SS, Zhou J, Wong PW, Kowalisyn J, Strokosch G. Intermediate homocysteinemia: a thermolabile variant of methylenetetrahydrofolate reductase. Am J Hum Genet. 1988; 43(4):414-21.

[103] Rees MM, Rodgers GM. Homocysteinemia: association of a metabolic disorder with vascular disease and thrombosis. Thrombosis Research. 1993; 71:337-359.

[104] Ubbink JB, Vermaak WJ, Van der Merwe A, Becker PJ. Vitamin B12, vitamin B6, and folate nutritional status in men with hyperhomocysteinemia. Am J Clin Nutr. 1993; 57:47-53.

[105] Mudd SH, Skovby F, Levy HL, Pettigrew KD, Wilcken B, Pyeritz RE et al. The natural history of homocystinuria due to cystathionine beta-synthase deficiency. Am J Hum Genet. 1985; 37:1-31.

[106] Engbertsen AMT, Franken DG, Boers GHJ, Stevens EMB, Grijbels FJM, Blom HJ. Thermolabile 5,10-methylenetetrahydrofolate reductase as a cause of mild hyperhomocysteinemia. Am J Hum Genet. 1995; 56:142-150.

[107] Frosst P, Blom HJ, Milos R, Goyette P, Sheppard CA, Matthews RG et al. A candidate genetic risk factor for vascular disease: a common mutation in methylenetetrahydrofolate reductase. Nat Genet. 1995; 10:111-113.

Chapter 2

Main Types of Clinical Appearance of Thrombophilic States During Pregnancy – Target Groups for Thrombophilia Testing

Ricardo Barini, Joyce Annichino-Bizzache,
Egle Couto, Marcelo Luis Nomura and
Isabela Nelly Machado

Additional information is available at the end of the chapter

1. Introduction

Normal pregnancy is associated with complex changes of hemostasis, leading to hypercoagulability states. Such physiological increase of blood coagulation during pregnancy occurs because of changes in the vascular endothelium and blood flow, generating changes from the 10th gestational week on. The changes may create a hypercoagulability state that results in thrombosis. The purpose of the hypercoagulability state during pregnancy is to prevent excessive bleeding by the time of delivery (Moreira, et al. 2008).

Normal hemostasis during pregnancy is the result of a balance between the system that promotes blood coagulation and the one inhibiting excessive coagulation (fibrinolytic system).

Gestational effects on coagulation proteins may be detected after the 3rd month of pregnancy, with significant changes in pro-coagulant proteins in comparison with physiological inhibitors. So, although changes in hemostatic system are intended for adaptation and protection of the pregnant woman's body, they may cause increased risk of thromboembolic events.

Despite of being physiological, excessive activation of the coagulation mechanism during pregnancy may lead to thromboembolic events, especially in women with hereditary and/or acquired factors who have a known predisposition to thrombi formation.

Thrombophilia is a hereditary or acquired disease related to changes in hemostasis mechanisms that are characterized by an increased trend to blood coagulation and consequent risk of thromboembolism (Machac S 2006). Hereditary factors that are considered potentially responsible for such trend to thrombosis are: protein C deficiency, protein S deficiency, anti-thrombin deficiency, presence of Factor V Leiden, a change in allele prothrombin 20210 G>A gene and a change in the gene of enzyme methylenetetrahydrofolate reductase (D'Amico 2006).

Thrombophilia hereditary causes have been researched since 1956, when Jordan and Nandorff introduced the term thrombophilia. In 1965 anti-thrombin deficiency was identified as the genetic cause of thrombophilia.

Such studies became larger in the 80's, when protein S and protein C deficiencies were described, as well as Factor V Leiden, in 1994. (Reistma PH 2007). Approximately 40% of thrombosis cases showing arterial occlusion or venous occlusion are hereditary. Venous thromboembolism frequently occurs as a result of several factors. Generally, thrombophilia should be seen as a multi-factorial disorder, not as the expression of a single genetic change (Buchholz T 2003).

The importance of angiogenesis for embryo implantation and the presence of thrombophilia leading to micro-thrombosis at the implantation site with subsequent impairment of embryo nidation and placental development should be considered as well (Vaquero E 2005).

The presence of thrombophilia was proven to be related to an increased risk of complications during pregnancy, such as pre-eclampsia, intrauterine growth restriction, premature detachment of placenta, preterm delivery, recurrent miscarriage, chronic fetal distress, besides ischemic events during pregnancy (Couto E 2005) (Ren A 2006) (Hoffman E 2012) (Bennet SA 2012).

Events related to thrombophilic changes during pregnancy are shown below.

2. Thrombophilia and pregnancy

One of the most important discussions in clinical practice regards the indication to search for a thrombophilic factor. This is due to elevated testing costs and its relevance to medical management once diagnose is done.

Access to Internet and available information on practically all matters brings up questioning by patients who look for these data regarding their personal risks and ask doctors how would they have to behave. It is an important role for doctors to help patients to discriminate which information are relevant for them, helping patient to pursue adequate options for personal treatment and prophylaxis.

There has been a great deal of research relating thrombophilia to many clinical situations where no scientific data is relevant. On the other side, there are still other clinical situations where there is no consensus, or even there will not be a practical condition to define a medical practice, based on studies performed up until now.

Women are exposed to a great variety of factors that increase their risk of venous thromboembolism (VTE) such as the use of hormonal contraception, pregnancy, puerperium and hormonal replacement therapy for menopause.

The incidence of VTE is higher in woman during pregnancy and post partum when compared to not pregnant women. There is an increase between five to ten times the risks of VTE, with an incidence of 0.6 to 1.3 events for 1.000 deliveries (Heit JA 2005) (McColl MD 1997).

Although there are controversies whether the occurrence of VTE is greater during pregnancy or post partum, it seems that this risk is equally distributed during all gestational period (Pomp ER 2008). VTE is the most important cause of maternal death (Marik PE 2008).

Hereditary thrombophilia include Factor V Leiden (FVL), G20210A prothrombin gene mutation, protein S, protein C and antithrombin III deficiency.

Prevalence of a hereditary thrombophilia is higher in women that had VTE during pregnancy, especially FVL and G20210A gene mutation. In Japanese populations, protein S seems to be the most common among pregnant women with VTE (Miyata T 2009).

Normal gestation is characterized by hypercoagulation, with increase of coagulation factors II, VII, IX, X, XII, fibrinogen and Von Willebrand factor. There is a reduction in natural anti coagulant factors, such as protein S, protein C and antithrombin III. There is also a reduction in fibrinolysis caused by reduction in tissue plasminogen activating factor (t-PA) and increase in the inhibitor of plasminogen activator (PAI-1). Increase of Factor VIII and reduction of protein S lead to a resistance to activated protein C. Thus, all these changes in pregnancy favor VTE.

After a VTE antecedent, thrombophilia is the most important individual risk factor for a new thrombotic episode during gestation.

Besides VTE, recurrent abortions and other complications during pregnancy can be associated to thrombophilia, particularly protein S deficiency and late complications.

A recent meta analysis has shown that a pregnant woman with thrombophilia has a greater risk than non pregnant woman, particularly in the presence of homozygosis to Leiden Factor V, to G20210A prothrombin gene mutation, in the presence of double heterozygosis for these two mutations and in the presence of antithrombin III deficiency. All of these thrombophilias, except MTHRF 677C>T gene mutation, even in homozygosis, bring about a statistically higher risk of VTE during pregnancy (Robertson L 2006).

The predictive value for the risk of VTE relating pregnancy and thrombophilia is described on table 1. (L. B. Pierangeli SS 2011).

Although, the absolut risk of VTE is low due to the low incidence of VTE itself. Even the risk of VTE in more severe thrombophilia, such as antithrombin III deficiency and protein S deficiency is low.

Thrombophilia	PPV*
FVL heterozygous state	1:500
prothrombin 20210 G>A heterozygous state	1:200
Double heterozygous state FVL + G20210A	4.6:100
Protein C deficiency	1:113
Antithrombin III deficiency	1:2.8
* PPV- positive predictive values	

Table 1. Predictive values of hereditary thrombophilias and VTE.

Medical management of pregnant women with thrombophilia will depend on the risk analysis; which may be complicated, because medical actions are based upon retrospective studies, meta-analysis or case control studies.

The evaluation of other risk factors for VTE, personal and familial VTE history (first degree relatives with VTE or arterial disease at age under fifty years old) should be taken into account seriously.

Hereditary thrombophilia can be classified in thee risk categories (Fogerty AE 2009):

- High risk: FVL homozygosis, prothrombin 20210 G>A gene mutation in homozygosis, double heterozygosis of FVL and prothrombin 20210 G>A, antithrombin III deficiency or any thrombophilia with a previous VTE.

- Intermediate risk: thrombophilia not classified as high risk with family history of VTE.

- Low risk: heterozygosis for FVL, for prothrombin 20210 G>A, protein C and protein S deficiency, lack of familial history or personal history for VTE.

As it is observed, personal or familial history of VTE has a strong weight on the VTE risk implication.

A pregnant woman with thrombophilia that presents with VTE during pregnancy has to be treated as a woman without thrombophilia with VTE. Treatment is based on heparin, particularly low molecular weight heparin, with doses adjusted by maternal weight. Warfarin can be exceptionally considered after the first trimester up till 34 weeks gestation. Fondaparinux has already been used in pregnant patients who were unable to use other heparin.

Anticoagulation is recommended for six weeks after delivery for all women with hereditary thrombophilia. During gestation, individual risk should be considered. Patients with high risk should receive heparin prophylaxis as a treatment doses or intermediate dose. Patients with intermediate risk should receive prophylactic heparin dose. Low risk patients should be followed up carefully with strict recommendations to look for medical assistance in the event of any symptoms that can be related to VTE.

Thrombophilia should be searched in any patient with familial history or personal history of VTE or with the diagnosis of a hereditary thrombophilia on a first degree relative.

A prospective study with 134 pregnant women heterozygous for FVL failed to show an increase in the incidence of VTE. Thus, although being the most common hereditary thrombophilia, its search is not to be indicated indiscriminately on every pregnant patient, nor prophylaxis is to be offered to asymptomatic carriers (Dizon-Townson D 2005).

A recently published meta-analysis including ten prospective studies showed only a small absolute risk for fetal death with demonstration of a small absolut risk with a smaller risk of fetal death on heterozygous FVL (Rodger MA 2010).

It is suggested based on the experience of many studies that generalized search for thrombophilia it is not indicated during pregnancy, except for patients with recent VTE event, or punctual search of a familial or personal in one family member. History of VTE is the most indicated event to look for thrombophilia.

Although thrombophilia are associated to an increase to the relative risk of complications during pregnancy, including VTE, the absolut risk is still low.

3. Clinical interferences of thrombophilia in pregnancy

Pregnancy by itself is considered a hypercoagulation state. Likewise for diabetes, it is expected to increase venous or arterial thromboembolism during pregnancy. The increase in estrogen levels leads to increase in many of the coagulation factors. Thus, in the presence of a hereditary or acquired thrombophilia a higher incidence of thrombotic events could be expected. Once a thrombophilic state is already identified, than we can expect a higher chance of clinical and obstetrical complications, except if prophylactic or therapeutic treatments are offered by caring physicians and followed by patients.

Although this is a disseminated belief, systematic reviews fail to demonstrate such strong relation. As stated above, only patients with a familial history of thrombosis or thrombophilia should be investigated.

However, this is not universally agreed on the literature. For instance, a group of patients with Leiden Factor V were compared to a group of absent mutation. It was observed that the group with the mutation had no thromboembolic events, whereas the group without had 2,7% thromboembolism (Dizon-Townson D 2005).

It has been also stated that even in relatives of probands who have no history of venous thromboembolism (VTE) should not receive antithrombotic prophylaxis during pregnancy because no difference was seen in the group with and without positive history of VTE prior to pregnancy (Cordoba I 2012). With theses considerations, one must look for evidences presented to date.

3.1. Thrombophilia and venous thromboembolism

Pregnancy is a clinical situation associated with increased risk of VTE, which increased from twofold to fourfold when these women presented a positive family history of VTE (Bezemer

ID 2009). Hereditary thrombophilia also increases the risk of VTE. However, the most important for prevention of thrombosis in pregnant women with these additive risk factors is the negative or positive history of previous VTE.

A meta-analysis and a review demonstrated increased risk of VTE in pregnant women with thrombophilia without a family or a positive history of VTE (Robertson L 2006) (Biron-Andreani C 2006). Heterozygosis for factor V Leiden and prothrombin 20210 G>A variant were fortunately associated with the lower risk, as they were the most common inherited thrombophilia. However, the homozygosis for these mutations was associated with the higher risk. Deficiencies of natural anticoagulants were also associated to increased risk of VTE.

The incidence of VTE in the pregnancy is 1/1,000 deliveries, and the absolute risk of VTE in thrombophilic women without a prior event or family history is in the range of 5-12/1,000 deliveries, except for homozygous carriers of the factor V Leiden or the prothrombin mutations, in whom the estimated baseline risk is about 4%.

Although the estimated risk of VTE in the presence of a positive family history of VTE and inherited thrombophilia without a previous episode of VTE has been described, it is imprecise, particularly for the rare thrombophilias (Friederich PW 1996).

Previous studies described higher risk of VTE in the presence of deficiencies of the anticoagulants, particularly antithrombin deficiency. However, methodological limitations could have contributed to these conclusions (Conard J 1990). The recent studies showed similar risks, even in double heterozygous for Leiden FV and prothrombin mutation (Tormene D 2001) (Martinelli I 2008). The homozygosis for MTHFR C>T alone does not lead to an increased risk of VTE in pregnant women (Robertson L 2006).

Women with thrombophilia without a family history presented a low risk of VTE. Because of the absence of high-quality evidence measuring the effectiveness and safety of antithrombotic agents in preventing VTE in patients with thrombophilia and a positive family history the recommendations have limitations.

The most recent guidelines suggest antepartum prophylaxis with prophylactic or intermediate-dose LMWH and postpartum prophylaxis for 6 weeks with prophylactic or intermediate-dose LMWH or vitamin K antagonists targeted at INR 2.0 to 3.0 for pregnant women with no prior history of VTE who are known to be homozygous for factor V Leiden or the prothrombin 20210 G>A mutation and have a positive family history for VTE (Bates SM and Physicians. 2012).

For patients with other thrombophilias without a previous history of VTE and who have a positive family history for VTE it is indicated antepartum clinical vigilance and postpartum prophylaxis for 6 weeks with prophylactic or intermediate dose LMWH or, in women who are not protein C or S deficient, vitamin K antagonists targeted at INR 2.0 to 3.0 (Bates SM and Physicians. 2012).

The same is indicated for pregnant women with no prior history of VTE who are known to be homozygous for factor V Leiden or the prothrombin 20210 G>A mutation and who do not have a positive family history for VTE (Bates SM and Physicians. 2012).

Pregnant women with all other thrombophilias and no prior VTE who do not have a positive family history for VTE, antepartum and postpartum clinical vigilance are indicated (Bates SM and Physicians. 2012).

3.2. Thrombophilia and arterial vascular accidents in pregnancy

Stroke in pregnancy is one of the main causes of maternal death and pregnancy and puerperium are known to increase its occurrence. The incidence of stroke is not precisely known and there is a wide variation among reports across the world, ranging from 1.5 to 69 per 100 thousand pregnancies (Jaigobin C 2000) (Scott CA 2012). Stroke accounts for 2.2% of all deaths in women of reproductive age and most of these deaths occur during pregnancy (WHO, 2004). Puerperium increases the risk of stroke 5-18-fold and cerebral thromboembolism carries a mortality rate 3 times higher in pregnant women. Despite the epidemiological association, stroke is considered a multifactorial disease, and genetic, environmental, vascular and hormonal factors play a complex and integrated role. Multiple genes have been studied, and even in the same individual, more than one polymorphism, acting in inflammatory, vascular and thrombotic pathways can lead to stroke.

With increasing worldwide efforts and acknowledgement to know about the causes and lessen the consequences of stroke, pregnant women seem to be a special population, not only because of the greater mortality but also because of the perinatal implications.

Obstetrical associated conditions are chronic hypertension, preeclampsia and cesarean delivery. However, most cases do not have predisposing factors and occur in apparently healthy subjects. Some physiologic changes during pregnancy and puerperium can be associated with an increased risk of stroke: increased circulating blood volume, increased cardiac output, vascular wall fragility, and high levels of steroid hormones.

Preeclampsia seems to be a risk factor even for non-pregnancy associated ischemic stroke, which means that women who had preeclampsia have an increased risk of, is when non-pregnant (Brown DW 2006). Non-obstetric risk factors include thrombophilia (inherited and acquired) migraine, smoking, advanced maternal age, diabetes, sickle cell disease, autoimmune conditions, and severe hypotension (Scott CA 2012).

Stroke in pregnancy and puerperium has three major clinical syndromes: ischemic stroke (IS), intracranial hemorrhage (ICH) and cerebral venous thrombosis (CVT). It is the most frequent presentation and CVT is rare. Maternal mortality can be as high as 50% for ICH and 20-25% overall (Nomura ML 2012) (Scott CA 2012).

There are few studies addressing the role of thrombophilia in stroke occurring during pregnancy or puerperium. We will focus mainly in thrombotic and ischemic stroke, since hemorrhagic stroke has different pathogenic mechanisms in pregnancy, mainly related to rupture of undiagnosed intracranial aneurysms and complications of eclampsia.

3.2.1. Inherited thrombophilia

Inherited thrombophilias can be found in up to 11 % of patients with stroke (Bushnell CD 2000). In this systematic review, no association was found between factor V Leiden and IS, but a slight increase in the odds ratio for prothrombin gene mutation was found (1.4; 95% CI 1.03-1.9).

A study by Voetsch (Voetsch B 2000) among 167 patients with ischemic stroke and did not find an association with inherited thrombophilia, except in cerebral venous thrombosis, where prothrombin gene mutation was more prevalent. For the small group of patients of African origin, homozygosis for MTHFR 677C>T might have a potential role. Interestingly, patients with CVT were all in use of oral contraceptives or in the puerperium.

Hankey (Hankey GJ 2001) tested 219 patients with ischemic stroke for inherited thrombophilia in a case-control study and did not find a significant association (prevalence of 14.7% in stroke patients and 11.7% in control subjects) between any thrombophilia or combination of thrombophilias and IS, and the authors conclude that routine testing is not recommended in the majority of patients.

Kim & Becker (Kim RJ 2003) performed a meta-analysis of the association between some inherited thrombophilias and ischemic stroke and factor V, prothrombin, and homocysteine metabolism were found to modestly increase the risk in young women.

Weber & Busch (Weber R 2005) performed a cost analysis of screening for inherited thrombophilias in patients with IS of unknown cause and concluded that screening was of questionable value, with the exception of antiphospholipid antibodies in younger patients.

Corod-Artal et al (Carod-Artal FJ 2005) screened 130 young patients with stroke, and only protein S deficiency was found to be associated with stroke of unknown cause in young subjects, but in this subpopulation 31% were oral contraceptive users.

Hamzi et al (Hamzi K 2011) performed the largest meta-analysis to date regarding possible genes associated with ischemic stroke, with more than 150 thousand subjects included. They found that MTHFR 677C>T, factor V Leiden, 20210 G>A prothrombin and ACE I/D polymorphism had significant, although very modest, associations with IS. However, the authors did not specify results in selected populations, such as pregnant women.

Haeusler et al (Haeusler KG 2012) reported an increased prevalence of factor VII polymorphisms and factor V Leiden (although not significant) in patients with cryptogenic (unknown cause) stroke.

All studies reported might have biases, such as selection of high-risk patients, and there is a lack of controlled, prospective studies in pregnant women. Recommendations for routine screening of inherited thrombophilias in the setting of stroke in pregnant or postpartum women cannot be made at present, since pregnancy itself might be the most important risk factor.

Inherited thrombophilia might play a role when associated with other conditions, acting synergistically or increasing the odds of other risk factors, such as puerperium (particularly in CVT), preeclampsia/eclampsia, oral contraceptive use and acquired thrombophilias, such as sickle cell disease.

3.2.2. Acquired thrombophilia

Acquired thrombophilia is a condition known to be associated with stroke. Transient cerebral ischemia and stroke (including CVT) are clinical manifestations of antiphospholipid syndrome (APS), but in order to establish the diagnosis a laboratory criteria must also be present, which might be detection in the plasma of lupus anticoagulant, or anticardiolipin antibodies (IgG or IgM) or anti-beta2-glycoprotein (IgG or IgM), in at least two occasions, 12 weeks apart, and according to specific standard laboratory guidelines (Miyakis S 2006). The association between IS and APS (primary and lupus-associated) is well established in case-control studies, and even in unselected populations this association seems strong (Bushnell CD 2000).

Patients with previous cerebrovascular events who met criteria for APS should have anti-thrombosis prophylaxis prescribed when pregnant, with non-fractioned or low-molecular weight heparin. Prophylaxis should be extended into 6 weeks postpartum also. Aspirin can also be added, particularly in the acute phase of an IS.

Patients with APS and previous cerebrovascular events have an increased recurrence risk of IS, and preeclampsia seems to be an additional risk factor (Fischer-Betz R 2012).

Other acquired thrombophilias or thrombophilic status can potentially increase the risk of stroke in pregnancy and puerperium, including sickle cell disease, nephrotic syndrome, dehydration or severe hypovolemic status, and careful attention must be paid in this situations.

4. Thrombophilia and pregnancy complications

Adverse pregnancy outcome are not infrequent in general population. Pregnancy complications include miscarriage, fetal loss, preeclampsia, fetal growth restriction, and placental abruption.

The association between inherited thrombophilic disorders and miscarriage, late fetal loss or severe preeclampsia has been described in various studies (Robertson L 2006) (v. d. Coppens M 2006) (Rodger MA 2010).

However, there is a high uncertainty about these associations, particularly for the less prevalent thrombophilia (Robertson L 2006). A meta-analysis including only prospective cohort studies showed only association between factor V Leiden and pregnancy loss, but not with other thrombophilias (Rodger MA 2010).

One randomized trial described increased live birth rate in women with factor V Leiden, the prothrombin gene mutation, or protein S deficiency using enoxaparin when compared with low-dose aspirin alone (Gris et al s et al), but the methodology was limited.

The results of other studies do not provide evidence that LMWH improves pregnancy outcome in women with inherited thrombophilia and recurrent pregnancy loss (F. N. Coppens M 2007).

Based on these findings the guidelines do not recommend screening for inherited thrombo-philia for women with a history of pregnancy complications. There is no indication of antith-rombotic prophylaxis for women with inherited thrombophilia and a history of pregnancy complications.

The results of two studies that address this issue, Heparin for Pregnant Women with Throm-bophilia [NCT01019655] and TIPPS: Thrombophilia in Pregnancy Prophylaxis Study [NCT00967382] are awaited with interest.

4.1. Thrombophilia and recurrent pregnancy loss

Pregnancy loss in humans occurs in up to 75% of fertilized ova and 15% of well-confirmed pregnancies (Boklage 1990) and recurrent pregnancy losses (RPL) affect 2–5% of women in reproductive age (Hatasaka 1994). RPL is usually defined as the loss of three or more consec-utive pregnancies before 20 weeks of gestation or with fetal weights less than 500 grams. Within this definition is a large and heterogeneous group of patients with many different causes of miscarriage. RPL frequency increases up to 5% when clinicians define RPL as two or more losses of pregnancy (Hogge 2003). In addition, epidemiological investigations have demon-strated that the frequency of subsequent pregnancy loss is 24% after two pregnancy losses, 30% after three and 40% after four successive pregnancy losses (Regan 1989). Additionally, recurrent risk for RPL may increase up to 50 percent even after six losses (Poland B 1977).

Recurrent abortion involves more than 500,000 women in the United States per year (Bick 2000). Within the past ten years interest in correlations between thrombophilia and complica-tions of pregnancy has remarkably increased. Thrombotic processes may also be involved in other serious obstetric complications, such as pre-eclampsia, intrauterine growth retardation and placental abruption by impairment of placental perfusion. Pregnancy itself induces a physiological hyper-coagulation state (Bick 2000) (Clark P 1998) (Stirling Y 1984) that might be aggravated by inherited or acquired thrombophilia. Results of studies on pregnancy complications in women with thrombophilia have been conflicting. This heterogeneous group of disorders results in increased venous and arterial thrombosis. Some thrombophilic states in RPL may be acquired such as antiphospholipid syndrome (APS) or heritable.

4.1.1. Acquired thrombophilia

Several studies have reported the presence of various autoantibodies in patients with RPL (Roussev RG 1996). However, only the antiphospholipid antibodies (APL) have been clearly associated to recurrent pregnancy losses both in patients with a known autoimmune disease, as APS or systemic lupus erythematous (SLE), and in the general population.

APL were thought to be directed against negatively charged phospholipids, but it has been shown that they are often directed against a protein cofactor, called beta 2 glycoprotein 1, that assists antibody association with the phospholipid (McNeil HP 1990). APL has been associated with thrombotic complications: some are systemic and some are pregnancy specific—sponta-neous abortion, stillbirth, intrauterine growth retardation, and preeclampsia (Harris 1986). Diagnosis of this syndrome requires at least one of each clinical and laboratory criterion

(ACOG 2005). Clinical criteria are: one or more confirmed episode of vascular thrombosis of any type (venous, arterial, small vessel) and/or pregnancy complications (three or more consecutive spontaneous pregnancy losses at less than 10 weeks of
gestation, one or more fetal deaths at greater than 10 weeks of gestation, one or more preterm births at less than 34 weeks of gestation secondary to severe
preeclampsia or placental insufficiency). Laboratory criteria are: positive plasma levels of anticardiolipin antibodies of the IgG or IgM isotope at medium to high levels and/or positive plasma levels of lupus anticoagulant. Testing must be positive on two or more occasions, 12 weeks or more apart (Miyakis S 2006).

The APS is the autoimmune disease most commonly associated with RPL (Rai RS 1995) to as low as 15% (Empson M 2002) and the presence of antiphospholipid antibodies is a major risk factor for an adverse pregnancy outcome (Out HJ 1992).

There is still controversy over the timing (early or late) of pregnancy loss more closely related with aPL. A retrospective study in a group of 366 women with recurrent pregnancy losses compared the type of prior pregnancy loss between women with and without APL (Oshiro et al, 1996). A total of 79 women included in the study tested positive for APL, while 290 did not. The rate of prior early pregnancy loss was similar in both groups (>80%). However, those patients with APL had 50% of prior late pregnancy losses compared with <25% late pregnancy loss rate in women without APL. The specificity of late pregnancy loss for the presence of APL was 76% compared with only 6% for two or more early pregnancy losses, thus suggesting that late pregnancy loss is the most frequent type of loss associated with APS. Other studies have found that most of the APL-related pregnancy losses were biochemical pregnancy losses or early pregnancy losses in nature (Parazzini F 1991) (MacLean MA 1994) (Yetman DL 1996). Experimental data using APS animal models further support the evidence that any type of pregnancy loss (including preimplantation embryos), but mainly embryo reabsorption, may be associated with APL (Ziporen L 1998).

The association of APL with recurrent pregnancy losses in patients with SLE and the APS suggests a causative role but, by no means, it does prove it. The major pregnancy-related target for APL is the placenta and utero-placental insufficiency is often attributed to vasculopathy of the terminal spiral arteries that nourish the placenta intervillous space. These vessels had smaller diameter and showed intimal lawyer thickening, fibrinoid necrosis, and intraluminal thrombosis (De Wolf et al, 1982). In other cases, the infarcted region may show villous congestion and hemorrhage and early trophoblastic necrosis (Bendon RW 1987). In addition to placental infarction and thrombosis, perivillous fibrin deposition and evidence of decidua vascular atherosis, indicative of spiral artery vasculopathy, are seen in some APS cases (Gharavi AE 2001).

The mechanisms by which aPL cause the above described changes are not completely under-stood and several hypotheses have been proposed. The earliest one is eicosanoid balance alteration mediated by aPL. Inhibition of endothelial cell production of PGI2 (a potent inhibitor of platelet aggregation and vasodilator) and enhancement of placental TXA2 production by plasma from aPL-positive women have been demonstrated by some investigators (Carreras LO 1981) (Schorer AE 1992). Another possible mechanism for thrombosis in APS is the cross-reactivity between APL and glycosaminoglycans, a family of heparin-like substances related with the non-thrombotic properties of the vascular endothelium. The inhibition of this function by APL may in part explain the thrombosis associated with them (Chamley LW 1993). Additionally, APL may interfere with the function of natural inhibitors of coagulation such as placental anticoagulant proteins (PAP) and others. PAP is a group of four calcium-dependent phospholipid-binding proteins that inhibit phospholipid- dependent steps of coagulation by making phospholipid inaccessible to clothing factors (Walker JH 1992). The major component of the PAP family is the PAP-1, also called annexin V, which is most abundant in the placenta. Annexin V and aPL compete for phospholipids in coagulation assays (Sammaritano LR 1992). It has been shown that distribution of annexin V over the intervillous surface was significantly lower in patients with APS that in women with recurrent pregnancy losses (Rand JH 1994). These findings suggest that reduced annexin V production and inhibition of its anticoagulant function by aPL may play a role in pregnancy loss in APS patients.

However, other non-thrombotic mechanisms have been implicated, being interference with the embryonic implantation the one that has received more attention. The APL have been found to react directly with third trimester villous trophoblastic cells (Lyden TW 1992) (Di Simone N 2000), prevent proliferation of trophoblast derived from choriocarcinoma cells (Chamley LW 1993), inhibit in vitro chemotaxis and differentiation of villous trophoblast isolated from third trimester placentae (Di Simone N 2000), decrease trophoblast invasion (Sebire NJ 2002) (Bose P 2005), and inhibit extra-villous trophoblast differentiation (Quenby S 2005). Furthermore, APL can induce pregnancy loss in mice by impairing the embryonic implantation capacity, likely because a direct interaction with the throphoectoderm cells (Sthoeger ZM 1993).

Additionally, aPL may impair the placenta production of chorionic gonadotropin during the early phases of pregnancy, thus determining the embryonic evolution (Shurtz-Swirski R 1993) and, in the mice model, APS is associated with a diminished secretion of interleukin-3, positively related with pregnancy the pregnancy loss is prevented by in vitro administration of recombinant interleukin-3 (Fishman P 1993).

Furthermore, the role of complement activation by the aPL has also received a great deal of attention. Several studies have suggested that activation of the complement cascade is necessary for aPL-mediated thrombophilia and fetal loss (G. G.-O. Pierangeli SS n.d.) (Holers VM 2002). It was found that inhibition of the complement cascade in vivo, using the C3 convertase inhibitor complement receptor 1-related gene protein y (Crry)-Ig, blocks aPL-induced fetal loss and growth retardation, and reversed aPL-mediated thrombosis (Holers VM 2002).

4.1.2. Inherited thrombophilia

In 1996 the first reports on an association between other forms of thrombophilia and recurrent pregnancy loss were published (Preston FE 1996) (Rai RS 1995) (Sanson BJ, 1996). Since then numerous case control studies investigating the impact of thrombophilia on pregnancy loss have been conducted (Kupferminc MJ 1999) (Gris JC R.-N. S., 1997) (Grandone E 1997) (Younis JS, 2000) (Pihusch R 2001) (Alonso A, 2002) (Rasmussen A, 2004). In most of these studies factor

V Leiden (Factor V 1691 G>A), prothrombin 20210 G>A and the methylene tetrahydrofolate gene 677 C>T variations were determined. Some studies also included other classical markers of thrombophilia, such as antithrombin III, protein C and protein S deficiency and APL (Kupferminc MJ 1999)(Kupferminc MJ, 1999) (Gris JC Q. I., 2000).

The normal coagulation pathway is pivotal for the pregnancy outcomes. Also any kind of disorder in coagulation pathway may cause thrombophilia that may be the reason of placental insufficiency and pregnancy loss (Reznikoff-Etievan MF, 2001). It has become clear that pro-thrombotic changes are associated with a substantial proportion of these fetal losses. Throm-bophilic defects, including mutations in factor V Leiden and prothrombin 20210 G>A, and deficiencies in protein C, protein S, and antithrombin III, have been reported in 49–65% of women with pregnancy complications and in 18–22% of women with normal pregnancies (B. 1999) (Kupferminc MJ, 1999).

Therefore, the role of thrombophilias in RPL has generated a great deal of interest. This heterogeneous group of disorders results in increased venous and arterial thrombosis. Although some thrombophilic states in RPL may be acquired such as APS, most are heritable such as hyperhomocyteinemia, activated protein C resistance, deficiencies in proteins C and S, mutations in prothrombin, and mutations in antithrombin III. The three most known common genetic markers for thrombophilia to predispose to venous thrombosis are; factor V Leiden (FVL), methylenetetrahydrofolate reductase mutation (MTHFR 677 C>T) and pro-thrombin gene mutation. Thrombophilic disorders have generated considerable interest in the field of RPL. Thrombophilia is an important predisposition to thrombosis due to a pro-coagulant state. Several blood-clotting disorders are grouped under the term of thrombophilia. Clinical studies suggest that the underlying pathophysiological mechanism is mediated via hypercoagulation, leading to utero-placental insufficiency with resultant pregnancy loss. The basis for the association between adverse fetal outcomes and heritable thrombophilias has focused on the mechanisms of impaired placental development and function secondary to venous or arterial thrombosis at the maternal–fetal interface (Aubard Y, 2000) (Cotter AM 2001) (Jeanine F, 2010).

Mutation in the gene-encoding factor V results in a protein that is resistant to the effects of activated protein C (aPC). The most common of a variety of mutations is at position 506 with a glutamine substitution for arginine; this FV: R506Q mutation is called the factor V Leiden mutation. The mutation results in a protein resistant to the effects of activated protein C (aPC). The net result is increased the cleavage of prothrombin to thrombin, which causes excessive coagulation.

The resistance to aPC has emerged as the commonest genetic cause of thromboembolism. It is caused by FVL in 95% of cases. The risk of thrombosis is increased 5- to 10-fold in heterozygous carriers of FVL, and 100-fold in homozygosis (Kovalevsky G, 2004).

Inherited decreased or absent antithrombin III activity will lead to increased thrombin formation and clotting. Prothrombin gene mutation is signaled by a defect in clotting factor II at position G20210A. The relative risk for thrombosis in patients with this mutation is two-fold in heterozygotes.

Individuals with hiperhomocisteinemia exhibit a deficiency of folate due to the presence of the methylene tetrahydrofolate reductase mutation (MTHRF 677C>T C677 T). The thrombotic risk is increased two-fold in homozygosis; and in the heterozygous state for Antithrombin III deficiency, the risk is 20- to 50-fold.

Consistent with general thrombotic risk, carriage of combinations of two or more inherited thrombophilic defects has particularly strong association with adverse pregnancy outcomes (Lockwood C. J., 2002) (Preston FE, 1996). Considerable attention has been directed recently toward a possible relationship between thrombophilias and certain pregnancy complications other than venous thrombosis (De Santis M, 2006).

4.1.3. In vitro fertilization failures and thrombophilia

The known or purported causality of phospholipid antibodies and coagulation factors on recurrent pregnancy loss long ago spilled over into the arena of conception with IVF or more precisely, the lack of it. Some have argued that without implantation to signal the arrival of an embryo, it would be improbable for serum or tissue-based response elements to prevent implantation. Others have argued that the effect is unrelated to the embryo, but rather the negative impact is at the level of the endometrium. The Practice Committee of the American Society for Reproductive Medicine released a Committee Opinion in 1999, which it reviewed again in 2008, ''Anti-phospholipid antibodies (APA) do not affect IVF success'' (Practice Committee of American Society for Reproductive Medicine. 2012). The review culled 16 peer-reviewed papers, of which 7 included appropriate endpoints and controls. There was no statistically significant impact of the presence of phospholipid antibodies on IVF outcomes neither when studies were examined individually nor when the data were aggregated in the 2,053 patients studied. The authors concluded that ''assessment of APA is not indicated among couples undergoing IVF. Therapy is not justified on the basis of existing data.''

A review was recently published on the topic of thrombophilias and IVF outcome (Di Nisio M, 2011). The authors' initial search yielded 694 studies. Case reports, editorials, reviews, meta-analyses, studies with inadequate outcomes, absence of thrombophilia/anti-phospholipid antibodies, and more than one of the above was excluded and 33 (6,092 patients) were ultimately analyzed. They report that twenty-nine studies (5,270 patients) assessed anti-phospholipid antibodies in women treated with assisted reproductive techniques (ART). The prevalence of antibodies in infertile patients varied from 0%–45%. When examining case-control studies, the authors write ''overall, the presence of one or more anti-phospholipid antibodies was associated with a 3-fold higher risk of ART failure.'' There was a significant degree of heterogeneity across these case-control studies.

4.2. Thrombophilia and fetal growth restriction

Obstetricians have been very interested on the possible consequences of thrombophilia because in face of an unexpected pregnancy event, such as fetal growth restriction not associated to preeclampsia or arterial hypertension, colagenosis as Systemic Lupus or any other maternal identified disease. This has been the casa once many patients that would have the profile for antiphospholipid syndrome showed no abnormal antibodies on their laboratory workup. So, there would be another group of women that would have another type of "coagulation disorder" that would have to be sorted out.

Considering the possibility that fibrin deposition on the maternal surface of the placenta may impair gas exchanges and nutritional elements between mother and fetus, the model of a thrombophilic induced placental insufficiency seems very attractive.

It has to be emphasized that most studies focus on the maternal aspect of maternal thrombosis in thrombophilia and less is regarded on the obstetrical and fetal complications of thrombophilia in pregnancy.

It has been shown by some authors that this association is found in case control study (Monari F, 2012), where all thrombophilias evaluated had a greater incidence within patients with history of fetal death and that Factor II 20210 G>A gene mutation had also a predictive value for previous fetal deaths in this study population.

Others contest this association when placental infarction is evaluated in comparison to abnormal placentation (Franco C 2011). In this study, no association was found between the presence of thrombophilia and histological findings of infarction.

One of us (R.B., personal communication not published) have observed instances where patients develop placental ultrasonography abnormal image - Grade II or III during second trimester – (Grannum PA, 1979) together with fetal growth restriction that demonstrated true catch up in fetal growth and sustained or regression in placental grade upon prophylactic low-dose heparin and aspirin regimen. In two occasions patients showed to be Leiden Factor heterozygous and Protein S deficiency.

One interesting study showed an increase in the frequency of patients with prothrombin gene mutation associated to IUGR and abruptio placentae (Kupferminc MJ, Peri H, Zwang E, Yaron Y, Wolman I, 2000).

Although randomized trial are still necessary to address the question whether treatment should be advised for women with diagnosed hereditary thrombophilia to prevent adverse pregnancy results, many authors agree that treatment ensures good results, like the one reported by results Kosar (Kosar A 2011). The live birth rate for treated patients was only 62%, even with treatment, which brings up de the consideration that this is really a high-risk obstetrical population.

One group showed that the institution of low-molecular-weight heparin to women with previous fetal growth restriction or pre eclampsia had a dramatic reduction on the recurrence of these events on subsequent pregnancies (Kupferminc, 2011).

When reviewing the literature one must be careful with the conclusions offered because most of the studies do not have a good enough large sample size to draw final conclusions.

This is the case of the Australian study comparing pregnancy results of women with and without inherited thrombophilia and positive pregnancy with pre eclampsia, fetal restriction, fetal death or placental abruption. Groups comprised 115 women on each arm and no difference on the frequency of thrombophilia in the group with and without adverse history. Now we have to wonder that for instance, Leiden Factor V is expected in less than 2% of any Caucasian population and 20210 G>A prothrombin gene mutation is even less frequent. A case control study would have to add up at least 600 hundred woman on each arm to be able to draw final conclusions.

A large cohort study of nulliparous women as performed where the results of inherited thrombophilia was blind to caring physicians and only a strong association of 20210 G>A prothrombin gene mutation was found to adverse results of their pregnancies (pre eclampsia, fetal death, fetal restriction, placenta abruption). None of the other thrombophilia showed association to any of these events in this asymptomatic population (Said, 2010).

When we look in the literature on acquired thrombophilia and fetal growth restriction, there is greater agreement that there is a relation between them.

4.3. Thrombophilia and preeclampsia

Preeclampsia is a leading cause of maternal-fetal morbidity and mortality. It accounts for a significant fraction of maternal deaths in developed and underdeveloped countries. Preeclampsia is one of the most researched diseases in medicine, and so far several aspects of its pathophysiology have been elucidated. However, a major concept that prevails among the most important studies is that preeclampsia is a multifactorial disease.

One of the most controversial aspects is the role of acquired and inherited thrombophilia in the development of preeclampsia. In this chapter, we present a review on the studies about thrombophilia and preeclampsia, with a critical standing point and future perspectives on this issue.

How thrombophilia might act as cause or contributor in preeclampsia? Thrombophilias may act as co-factor in decreasing placental function through vascular thrombosis and also may regulate inflammatory pathways and increase intravascular coagulation. Alltogether with other contributors these features may trigger endothelial dysfunction and lead to the clinical and laboratorial picture of preeclampsia (Kupferminc., 2003).

4.3.1. Inherited thrombophilias

Among inherited thrombophilias, the most studied are factor V Leiden mutation, 20210 G>A prothrombin mutation, MTHRF 677C>T, protein C deficiency, protein S deficiency and activated protein C resistance.

There are conflicting results regarding the association between inherited thrombophilias and preeclampsia. This might be due to several factors: small sample sizes, poor methodological quality, retrospective nature of most studies and heterogeneity in the prevalence of thrombophilia in different populations.

Initial reports showed a marked increase in the prevalence of thrombophilic mutations in women with preeclampsia compared to women with uneventful pregnancies, with figures of 40% to 72% for at least one mutation (Stella CL, 2006) (Kupferminc MJ, 1999). These studies were in most part case-control and included women with late and early-onset, mild and severe preeclampsia, as also HELLP syndrome and eclampsia.

Despite these convincing evidences, several studies further did not confirm such a strong association (Rodger, 2007).

Kosmas et al (Kosmas, 2003) reported a meta-analysis of more than 5,000 women among 19 studies. For the studies published until 2000, an association was found between factor V Leiden and preeclampsia, however, for the studies published in 2001-2002 this association was not confirmed.

Dizon-Towson et al (Dizon-Townson D, 2005) also found no association between factor V Leiden and prothrombin mutations with preeclampsia, and this was a multi-center, prospective study.

Another prospective study (Said, 2010) involving 2034 women did not find significant associations between any inherited thrombophilia and preeclampsia and the authors concluded that the majority of women with inherited thrombophilia have normal pregnancy outcomes.

Alfirevic et al. (Alfirevic, 2002) reported the first systematic review of the association between maternal thrombophilia and preeclampsia, and factor V Leiden mutation (heterozygous), 20210 G>A prothrombin mutation (heterozygous), MTHFR 677C>T (homozygous), protein C deficiency, protein S deficiency and activated protein C resistance were more prevalent among women with preeclampsia.

In a systematic review performed by Robertson et al. (Robertson L, 2006), the odds ratios for several genetic mutations (factor V Leiden, prothrombin mutation, MTHFR 677C>T and protein S) ranged from 1.37 to 3.49, with evidence of heterogeneity among some studies.

In a systematic review and meta-analysis, Rodger et al. (Rodger MA, 2010) failed to show a significant association between factor V Leiden and prothrombin gene mutation. This review included ten prospective cohort studies and more than twenty thousand patients.

Combined thrombophilias (being carrier of more than one mutation) might have a stronger association with early-onset, severe preeclampsia and HELLP syndrome, however conclusive and solid evidence is also lacking.

The American College of Obstetricians and Gynecologists (Lockwood C, Wendel G; Committee on Practice Bulletins— Obstetrics., 2011) stated that the evidence is insufficient to conclude that inherited thrombophilia increases the occurrence of preeclampsia and therefore do not recommend screening and treatment for thrombophilia in women with previous preeclampsia.

Lockwood (Lockwood C., 2010) also cautioned against screening and treatment for inherited thrombophilias, unless in the setting of a clinical trial. The author argues that methodological quality of the positive associations is questionable, that these associations are modest (3-fold increase) and that large prospective cohort studies did not show a consistent association.

In summary, the most recent evidence points to a weak association between preeclampsia and inherited thrombophilias. Even this evidence derives from small studies, with possible selection and report biases. The recent evidence also discourages treatment with heparin based on a diagnosis of inherited thrombophilia.

4.3.2. Acquired thrombophilia

Antiphospholipid antibodies are more frequently encountered in patients with preeclampsia, and in this setting they might be a modulator of the severity of the disease rather than a direct cause.

The Sydney Consensus Statement on Investigational Classification Criteria for the Antiphospholipid Syndrome (Miyakis S, 2006) included eclampsia or severe preeclampsia leading to preterm delivery prior to the 34th week as clinical criteria. To establish the diagnosis of antiphospholipid syndrome (APS) a laboratory criteria must also be present, which might be detection in the plasma of lupus anticoagulant, or anticardiolipin antibodies (IgG or IgM) or anti-beta2-glycoprotein (IgG or IgM), in at least two occasions, 12 weeks apart, and according to specific standard laboratory guidelines.

Do Prado et al (do Prado AD, 2010) performed a systematic review on the association between preeclampsia and anticardiolipin antibodies. The authors found a significant association with an odds ratio of 11.15 for severe preeclampsia and 2.86 for preeclampsia.

Abou-Nassar et al. (Abou-Nassar K, 2011) Published a systematic review of antiphospholipid antibodies and preeclampsia and found an inconsistent association, detected only in case-control studies but not in cohort studies, and of lower magnitude.

Although controversial, recent evidence suggests that treatment with heparin and low-dose aspirin in order to reduce recurrence risk is warranted in this situation, with overall pregnancy success rates of more than 70% (Ernest JM, 2011) (Lockwood C., 2010).

It must also be noted that women with APS are at greater risk of thromboembolism, and anticoagulation should be prescribed for this purpose also.

Author details

Ricardo Barini, Joyce Annichino-Bizzache, Egle Couto, Marcelo Luis Nomura and Isabela Nelly Machado

Faculdade de Ciências Médicas UNICAMP, SP, Brazil

References

[1] Abou-Nassar K, Carrier M, Ramsay T, Rodger MA. "The association between anti-phospholipid antibodies and placenta mediated complications: a systematic review and meta-analysis." Thromb Res 128, no. 1 (Jul 2011): 77-85.

[2] ACOG. "Antiphospholipid syndrome." Practice Bulletin No. 68, Nov 2005.

[3] Alfirevic, Z., Roberts, D., Martlew, V. "How strong is the association between maternal thrombophilia and adverse pregnancy outcome? A systematic review." Eur J Obstet Gynecol Reprod Biol, Feb 2002: 6-14.

[4] Alonso A, Soto I, Urgelles MF, Corte JR, Rodriguez MJ, Pinto CR. "Acquired and inherited thrombophilia in women with unexplained fetal losses." Am J Obstet Gynecol, 2002: 1337 - 42.

[5] Aubard Y, et al. "Hyperhomocysteinema and pregnancy review of our present understanding and therapeutic implications." Eur J Obstet Gynecol, 2000: 157–65.

[6] B., Brenner. "Inherited thrombophilia and pregnancy loss." Thromb Haemost, 1999: 634–640.

[7] Bates SM, Greer IA, Middeldorp S, Veenstra DL, Prabulos AM, Vandvik PO, and American College of Chest Physicians. "VTE, thrombophilia, antithrombotic therapy, and pregnancy: Antithrombotic Therapy and Prevention of Thrombosis, 9th ed: American College of Chest Physicians Evidence-Based Clinical Practice Guidelines." Chest. 141, no. 2 Suppl (Feb 2012): e691S-736S.

[8] Bendon RW, Wilson J, Getahun B, van der Bel-Kahn J. "A maternal death due to thrombotic disease associated with anticardiolipin antibody." Arch Pathol Lab, 1987: 370–372.

[9] Bennet SA, Bagot CN, Arya R. "Pregnancy loss and thrombophilia: the elusive link." Br J Haematol 157 (2012): 529-42.

[10] Bezemer ID, van der Meer FJ, Eikenboom JC, Rosendaal FR, Doggen CJ. "The value of family history as a risk indicator for venous thrombosis." Arch Intern Med 169 (2009): 610 - 615.

[11] Bick, R L. "Recurrent miscarriage syndrome due to blood coagulation protein/platelet defects: prevalence, treatment and outcome results. DRW Metroplex Recurrent Miscarriage Syndrome Cooperative Group." Clin Appl Thromb Hemost 6 (2000): 115-25.

[12] Biron-Andreani C, Schved JF, Daures JP. "Factor V Leiden mutation and pregnancy-related venous thromboembolism:what is the exact risk? Results from a meta-analysis." Thromb Haemost 18, no. 96 (2006): 14-18.

[13] Boklage, CE. "Survival probability of human conceptions from fertilization to term." Int J Fertil 35, no. 2 (Mar-Apr 1990): 75, 79-80, 81-94.

[14] Bose P, Black S, Kadyrov M et al. "Heparin and aspirin attenuate placental apoptosis in vitro: implications for early pregnancy failure." Am J Obstet Gynecol, 2005: 23–30.

[15] Brown DW, Dueker N, Jamieson DJ, Cole JW, Wozniak MA, Stern BJ, Giles WH, Kittner SJ. "Preeclampsia and the risk of ischemic stroke among young women: results from the Stroke Prevention in Young Women Study." Stroke 37, no. 4 (Apr 2006): 1055-9.

[16] Buchholz T, Thaler CJ. "Inherited Thrombophilia: Impact in Human Reproduction." Am J Reprod Immunol 50 (2003): 20-32.

[17] Bushnell CD, Goldstein LB. "Diagnostic testing for coagulopathies in patients with ischemic stroke." Stroke 31, no. 12 (2000): 3067-78.

[18] Carod-Artal FJ, Nunes SV, Portugal D, Silva TV, Vargas AP. "Ischemic stroke subtypes and thrombophilia in young and elderly Brazilian stroke patients admitted to a rehabilitation hospital." Stroke 36, no. 9 (2005): 2012-4.

[19] Carreras LO, Defreyn G, Machin SJ et al. "Arterial thrombosis, intrauterine death and "lupus" antiocoagulant: detec- tion of immunoglobulin interfering with prostacyclin formation." Lancet, 1981: 244–246.

[20] Chamley LW, McKay EJ, Pattison NS. "Inhibition of heparin/antithrombin III cofactor activity by anticardiolipin anti-bodies: a mechanism for thrombosis." Thromb Res, 1993: 103–11.

[21] Clark P, Brennand J, Conkie JA, McCall F, Greer IA, Walker ID. "Activated protein C sensitivity, protein C, protein S and coagulation in normal pregnancy.." Thromb Haemost 79 (1998): 1166 - 70.

[22] Conard J, Horellou MH, Van Dreden P, Lecompte T, Samama M. "Thrombosis and pregnancy in congenital deficiencies in AT III, protein C or protein S: study of 78 women." Thromb Haemost 63 (1990): 319 - 320.

[23] Coppens M, Folkeringa N, Teune M, et al. "Natural course of the subsequent pregnancy after a single loss in women with and without the factor V Leiden or prothrombin 20210A mutations." J Thromb Haemost 5 (2007): 1444-1448.

[24] Coppens M, van de Poel MH, Bank I, et al. "A prospective cohort study on the absolute incidence of venous thromboembolism and arterial cardiovascular disease in asymptomatic carriers of the prothrombin 20210A mutation." Blood 108 (2006): 2604 - 2607.

[25] Cordoba I, Pegenaute C, González-López TJ, Chillon C, Sarasquete ME, Martin-Herrero F, Guerrero C, Cabrero M, Garcia Sanchez MH, Pabon P, Lozano FS, Gonzalez M, Alberca I, González-Porras JR). "Risk of placenta-mediated pregnancy complications or pregnancy-related VTE in VTE-asymptomatic families of probands with VTE and heterozygosity for factor V Leiden or G20210 prothrombin mutation." Eur J Haematol 8, no. 3 (Sep 2012): 250-5.

[26] Cotter AM, et al. "Elevated plasma homocysteine in early pregnancy: A risk factor for the development of severe preeclampsia." Am J Obstet Gynecol, 2001: 781–5.

[27] Couto E, Nomura ML, Barini R, Silva JL. "Pregnancy- associated venous thromboembolism in combined heterozygous factor V Leiden and prothrombin G2022110A mutations." São Paulo Med J. 123 (2005): 286-88.

[28] De Santis M, et al. "Inherited and acquired thrombophilia: Pregnancy outcome and treatment." Reprod Toxicol, 2006: 227.

[29] Di Nisio M, Rutjes AWS, Ferrante N, Tiboni GM, Cuccurullo F, Porreca E. "Thrombophilia and outcomes of assisted reproduction technologies: a sys- tematic review and meta-analysis." Blood, 2011: 2670–8.

[30] Di Simone N, Meroni PL, Del Papa N et al. " Antiphospholipid antibodies affect trophoblast gonadotrophin secretion through adhered beta-2-glycoportein I." Arthritis Rheum, 2000: 140–50.

[31] D'Amico, EA. Trombofilia. Edited by Lorenzi TF. Rio de Janeiro, RJ: Guanabara Koogan;, 2006.

[32] Dizon-Townson D, Miller C, Sibai B, et al. "The relationship of the Factor V Leiden mutation in pregnancy outcomes for mother and fetus." Obstet Gynecol 106 (2005): 517–24.

[33] do Prado AD, Piovesan DM, Staub HL, Horta BL. "Association of anticardiolipin antibodies with preeclampsia: a systematic review and meta-analysis." Obstet Gynecol 116, no. 6 (Dec 2010): 1433-43.

[34] Empson M, Lassere M, Craig JC, Scott J. "Recurrent pregnancy loss with antiphospholipid antibody: a systematic review of therapeutic trials." Obstet Gynecol, 2002: 135–144.

[35] Ernest JM, Marshburn PB, Kutteh WH. "Obstetric antiphospholipid syndrome: an update on pathophysiology and management." Semin Reprod Med. 29, no. 6 (Nov 2011): 522-39.

[36] Fischer-Betz R, Specker C, Brinks R, Schneider M. "Pregnancy outcome in patients with antiphospholipid syndrome after cerebral ischaemic events: an observational study." Lupus 21, no. 11 (2012): 1183-9.

[37] Fishman P, Falach-Vaknine E, Zigelman R et al. "Prevention of fetal loss in experimental anti-phospholipid syndrome by in vitro administration of recombinant interleukin-3." J Clin Invest, 1993: 1834–77.

[38] Fogerty AE, Connors JM. "Management of inherited thrombophilia in pregnancy." Curr Opin Endocrinol Diabetes Obes 16 (2009): 464–9.

[39] Franco C, Walker M, Robertson J, Fitzgerald B, Keating S, McLeod A, Kingdom JC. "Placental infarction and thrombophilia." Obstet Gynecol, Apr 2011: 929-34.

[40] Friederich PW, Sanson BJ, Simioni P, et al. "Frequency of pregnancy-related venous thromboembolism in anticoagulant factor-deficient women: implications for prophylaxis." Ann Intern Med 125 (1996): 955 - 960.

[41] Gharavi AE, Pierangeli SS, Harris EN. "Mechanisms of pregnancy loss in antiphospholipid syndrome." Clin Obstet Gynecol, 2001: 11–19.

[42] Grandone E, Margaglione M, Colaizzo D, et al. "Factor V Leiden is associated with repeated and recurrent unexplained fetal losses." Thromb Haemost, 1997: 822 - 4.

[43] Grannum PA, Berkowitz RL, Hobbins JC. "The ultrasonic changes in the maturing placenta and their relation to fetal pulmonic maturity." Am J Obstet Gynecol 133, no. 8 (Apr 1979): 915-22.

[44] Gris JC, Quere I, Sanmarco M, et al. "Antiphospholipid and antiprotein syndromes in non-thrombotic, non- autoimmune women with unexplained recurrent primary early foetal loss. The Nimes Obstetricians and Haematologists Study NOHA." Thromb Haemost, 2000: 228 - 36.

[45] Gris JC, Ripart-Neveu S, Maugard C, et al. "Respective evaluation of the prevalence of haemostasis abnormalities in unexplained primary early recurrent miscarriages. The Nimes Obstetricians and Haematologists (NOHA) Study." Thromb Haemost, 1997: 1096 - 103.

[46] Haeusler KG, Herm J, Hoppe B, Kasabov R, Malzahn U, Endres M, Koscielny J, Jungehulsing GJ. "Thrombophilia screening in young patients with cryptogenic stroke. Prevalence of gene polymorphisms compared to healthy blood donors and impact on secondary stroke prevention." Hamostaseologie 32, no. 2 (2012): 147-52.

[47] Hamzi K, Tazzite A, Nadifi S. "Large-scale meta-analysis of genetic studies in ischemic stroke: Five genes involving 152,797 individuals." Indian J Hum Genet 17, no. 3 (2011): 212-7.

[48] Hankey GJ, Eikelboom JW, van Bockxmeer FM, Lofthouse E, Staples N, Baker RI. "Inherited thrombophilia in ischemic stroke and its pathogenic subtypes." Stroke 32, no. 8 (2001): 1793-9.

[49] Harris, EN. "Syndrome of the black swan." Br J Rheumatol 26 (1986): 324–326.

[50] Hatasaka, H H. "Recurrent miscarriage: epidemiologic factors, definitions and incidence." Clin Obstet Gynecol 37 (1994): 325–334.

[51] Heit JA, Kobbervig CE, James AH, Petterson TM, Bailey KR, Melton LJ III. "Trends in the incidence of venous thromboembolism during pregnancy or postpartum: a 30-year population based study." Ann Intern Med. 143 (2005): 697–706.

[52] Hoffman E, Hedlund E, Perin T, Lyndrup J. Is thrombophilia a risk factor for placenta – mediated pregnancy complications? Vol. 286. 3 vols. Arch Gynecol Obstet, 2012.

[53] Hogge, WA. et al. "The clinical use of karyotyping spontaneous abortions." Am. J. Obstet. Gynecol. 189 (2003): 397–400.

[54] Holers VM, Girardi G, Mo L et al. "C3 activation is required for anti-phospholipid antibody-induced fetal loss." J Exp Med, 2002: 211–220.

[55] Jaigobin C, Silver FL. "Stroke and pregnancy." Stroke 31, no. 12 (Dec 2000): 2948-51.

[56] Jeanine F, et al. "Prenatal Screening for Thrombophilias: Indications and Controversies." Clin Lab Med, 2010: 747–760.

[57] Kim RJ, Becker RC. "Association between factor V Leiden, prothrombin G20210A, and methylenetetrahydrofolate reductase C677T mutations and events of the arterial circulatory system: a meta-analysis of published studies." Am Heart J. 146, no. 6 (2003): 948-57.

[58] Kosar A, Kasapoglu B, Kalyoncu S, Turan H, Balcik OS, Gümüs EI. "Treatment of adverse perinatal outcome in inherited thrombophilias: a clinical study." Blood Coagul Fibrinolysis, Jan 2011: 14-8.

[59] Kosmas, IP., Tatsioni, A., Ioannidis, JP. "Association of Leiden mutation in factor V gene with hypertension in pregnancy and pre-eclampsia: a meta-analysis." J Hypertens, Jul 2003: 1221-8.

[60] Kovalevsky G, et al. "Evaluation of the association between hereditary thrombophilias and recurrent pregnancy loss: a meta-analysis." Arch Intern Med, 2004: 558-63.

[61] Kupferminc MJ, Eldor A, Steinman N, et al. "Increased frequency of genetic thrombophilia in women with complications of pregnancy." N Engl J Med, 1999: 9-13.

[62] Kupferminc MJ, Peri H, Zwang E, Yaron Y, Wolman I,. "High prevalence of the prothrombin gene mutation in women with intrauterine growth retardation, abruptio placentae and second trimester loss." Acta Obstet Gynecol Scand, Nov 2000: 963-7.

[63] Kupferminc, MJ. Rimon, E. Many, A. Sharon, M. Lessing, JB, Gamzu, R.. "Low molecular weight heparin treatment during subsequent pregnancies of women with inherited thrombophilia and previous severe pregnancy complications." J Matern Fetal Neonatal Med, Aug 2011: 1042-5.

[64] Kupferminc., MJ. "Thrombophilia and pregnancy." Reprod Biol Endocrinol., Nov 2003: 111.

[65] Lockwood C, Wendel G; Committee on Practice Bulletins— Obstetrics. "Practice Bulletin No. 124: Inherited thrombophilias in pregnancy. American College of Obstetricians and Gynecologists Committee on Practice Bulletins-Obstetrics." Obstet Gynecol, Sept 2011: 730-40.

[66] Lockwood, C J. "Inherited thrombophilias in pregnant patients: detection and treatment paradigm." Obstet Gynecol, 2002: 333–341.

[67]   Lockwood, C J. "Inherited thrombophilias in pregnant patients." Prenat Neonat Med, 2001: 3–14.

[68]   Lockwood, C.J. 2010. http://www.modernmedicine.com/modernmedicine/Modern +Medicine+Now/Stop-screening-for-inherited-thrombophilias-in-pat/ArticleStan- dard/Article/detail/668547 (accessed Sept 17, 2012).

[69]   Lyden TW, Vogt E, Ng AK, Johnson PM, Rote NS. "Monoclonal antiphospholipid an- tibody reactivity against human placental trophoblast." J Reprod Immunol, 1992: 1– 14.

[70]   Machac S, Lubusky M, Prochazka M, Streda R. "Prevalece of inherited thrombophilia in patients with severe ovarian hyperstimulation syndrome." Biomed Pap Med Fac Univ Palacky Olomouc Czech Repub. 150, no. 2 (2006): 289-292.

[71]   MacLean MA, Cumming GP, McCall F, Walker ID, Walker JJ. "The prevalence of lu- pus anticoagulant and anticardiolipin antibodies in women with a history of first tri- mester miscarriages." Br J Obstet Gynaecol, 1994: 103–106.

[72]   Marik PE, Plante LA. "Venous thromboembolic disease and pregnancy." N Engl J Med. 359 (2008): 2025–33.

[73]   Martinelli I, Battaglioli T, De Stefano V, et al. "GIT (Gruppo Italiano Trombofilia). The risk of fi rst venous Tromboembolism during pregnancy and puerperium in double heterozygotes for factor V Leiden and prothrombin G20210A." J Thromb Hae- most 6 (2008): 494 - 498.

[74]   McColl MD, Ramsay JE, Tait RC, Walker ID, McCall F, Conkie JA, et al. "Risk factors for pregnancy associated venous thromboembolism." Thromb Haemost. 78 (1997): 1183–8.

[75]   McNeil HP, et al. "Anti-phospholipid antibodies are directed against a complex anti- gen that includes a lipid binding inhibitor of coagulation: beta 2-glycoprotein I (apo- lipoprotein H).." Proc Natl Acad Sci U S A 87 (1990): 4120–4124.

[76]   Miyakis S, Lockshin MD, Atsumi T, Branch DW, Brey RL, Cervera R, Derksen RH, DE Groot PG, Koike T, Meroni PL, Reber G, Shoenfeld Y, Tincani A, Vlachoyianno- poulos PG, Krilis SA. "International consensus statement on an update of the classifi- cation criteria for definite antiphospholipid syndrome (APS)." J Thromb Haemost 4, no. 2 (2006): 295-306.

[77]   Miyata T, Sato Y, Ishikawa J, Okada H, Takeshita S, Sakata T, et al. "Prevalence of genetic mutations in protein S, protein C and antithrombin genes in Japanese pa- tients with deep vein thrombosis." Thromb Res. 124 (2009): 14–8.

[78]   Monari F, Alberico S, Avagliano L, Cetin I, Cozzolino S, Gargano G, Marozio L, Me- cacci F, Neri I, Tranquilli AL, Venturini P, Facchinetti F. "Relation between maternal thrombophilia and stillbirth according to causes/associated conditions of death." Ear- ly Hum Dev., Apr 2012: 251-4.

[79] Moreira, C.E.S.1, M.A.S.1 Ogino, A.C.R.2 de Moraes, and T.J.C. Neiva. "Hemostasia na gravidez estudo prospectivo RBAC." RBAC 42, no. 2 (2008): 111-113.

[80] Nomura ML, Olivares C, Min L L. "Stoke in pregnacy and puerperium: a Brazilian case series." Personal data, unpublished. 2012.

[81] Oshiro BT, Silver RM, Scott JR, Yu H, Branch DW. "Antiphospholipid antibodies and fetal death." Obstet Gynecol, 1996: 489–493.

[82] Out HJ, et al. " A prospective, controlled multicenter study of the obstetric risks of pregnant women with antiphospholipid antibodies." Br J Obstet Gynaecol, 1992: 26–32.

[83] Parazzini F, Acaia B, Faden D, Lovotti M, Marelli G, Cortelazzo S. "Antiphospholipid antibodies and recurrent abortion." Obstet Gynecol, Jun 1991: 854-8.

[84] Pierangeli SS, Girardi G, Vega-Ostertag M, Liu X, Espinola RG, Salmon J. "Requirement of activation of complement C3 and C5 for antiphospholipid antibody-mediated thrombophilia." Arthritis Rheum., Jul 2005: 2120-4.

[85] Pierangeli SS, Girardi G, Vega-Ostertag ME, Liu X, Espinola RG, Salmon J. "Requirement of activation of complement C3 and C5 for antiphospholipid antibody-mediated thrombophilia." Arthritis Rheum, 2120–2124.

[86] Pierangeli SS, Leader B, Barilaro G, Willis R, Branch DW. Acquired and inherited thrombophilic disorders in pregnancy. Vol. 38. Obstet Gynecol Clin N Am, 2011.

[87] Pihusch R, Buchholz T, Lohse P, et al. "Thrombophilic gene mutations and recurrent spontaneous abortion: prothrombin mutation increases the risk in the first trimester." Am J Reprod Immunol, 2001: 124 - 31.

[88] Poland B, et al. "Reproductive counseling in patients who have had a spontaneous abortion." Am J Obstet Gynecol, 1977: 127: 685.

[89] Pomp ER, Lenselink AM, Rosendaal FR, Doggen CJ. "Pregnancy, the postpartum period and prothrombotic defects: risk of venous thrombosis in the MEGA study." J Thromb Haemost. 6 (2008): 632–7.

[90] Practice Committee of American Society for Reproductive Medicine. "Diagnostic evaluation of the infertile female: a committee opinion." Fertil Steril, Aug 2012: 302-7.

[91] Preston FE, Rosendaal FR, Walker ID, et al. "Increased fetal loss in women with heritable thrombophilia." Lancet, 1996: 913-6.

[92] Quenby S, Mountfield S, Cartwright JE, Whitley GS, Chamley L, Vince G. "Antiphospholipid antibodies precent extravillous trophoblast differentiation.." Fertil Steril, 2005: 691–8.

[93]   Rai RS, Clifford K, Cohen H, Regan L. "High prospective fetal loss rate in untreated pregnancies of women with recurrent miscarriage and antiphospholipid antibodies." Hum Reprod, 1995: 3301–3304.

[94]   Rand JH, Wu XX, Guller S et al. "Reduction of annexin-V (placental anticoagulant protein-I) on placental villi of women with antiphospholipid antibodies and recurrent spontaneous abortion." Am J Obstet Gynecol, 1994: 1566–72.

[95]   Rasmussen A, Ravn P. "High frequency of congenital thrombophilia in women with pathological pregnancies?" Acta Obstet Gynecol Scand, 2004: 808 - 17.

[96]   Regan, L. et al. "Influence of past reproductive performance on risk of spontaneous abortion." BMJ 299 (1989): 541–545.

[97]   Reistma PH, Rosendaal FR. "Past and future of genetic research in thrombosis." J Thromb Haemost 5 (2007): 264-9.

[98]   Ren A, Wang J. "Methylenehydrofolate reductase C677T polymorphism and the risk of unexplained recurrent pregnancy loss: a meta-analysis." Fertility and Sterility 86 (2006): 1716-22.

[99]   Reznikoff-Etievan MF, et al. "Factor V Leiden and G20210A prothrombin mutations are risk factors for very early recurrent miscarriage." BJOG, 2001: 1251 - 1254.

[100] Robertson L, Wu O, Langhorne P, Twaddle S, Clark P, Lowe GD, Walker ID, Greaves M, Brenkel I, Regan L, Greer IA. "Thrombosis: Risk and Economic Assessment of Thrombophilia Screening (TREATS) Study.Thrombophilia in pregnancy: a systematic review." Br J Haematol 132, no. 2 (Jan 2006): 171–96.

[101] Rodger MA, Betancourt MT, Clark P, et al. "The association of factor V Leiden and prothrombin gene mutation and placenta-mediated pregnancy complications: a systematic review and meta-analysis of prospective cohort studies." PLoS Med 7, no. 6 (2010): e1000292.

[102] Rodger, MA., Paidas, M. "Do thrombophilias cause placenta-mediated pregnancy complications?" Semin Thromb Hemost, Sep 2007: 597-603.

[103] Roussev RG, Kaider BD, Price DE, Coulam CB. "Laboratory evaluation of women experiencing reproductive failure." Am J Reprod Immunol 35 (1996): 415–420.

[104] Said JM, Higgins JR, Moses EK, Walker SP, Monagle PT, Brennecke SP. "Inherited thrombophilias and adverse pregnancy outcomes: a case-control study in an Australian population." Acta Obstet Gynecol Scand, Feb 2012: 250-5.

[105] Said, JM., Higgins, JR., Moses, EK., Walker, SP., Borg, AJ., Monagle, PT., Brennecke, SP. "Inherited thrombophilia polymorphisms and pregnancy outcomes in nulliparous women." Obstet Gynecol, Jan 2010: 5-13.

[106] Sammaritano LR, Gharavi AE, Soberano C, Levy RA, Lockshin MD. "Phospholipid binding of antiphospholipid antibodies and placental anticoagulant protein." J Clin Immunol, 1992: 27–35.

[107] Sanson BJ, Friederich PW, Simioni P, et al. "The risk of abortion and stillbirth in antithrombin-, protein C-, and protein S-deficient women." Thromb Haemost, 1996: 387 - 8.

[108] Schorer AE, Duane PG, Woods VL, Niewoehner DE. "Some antiphospholipid antibodies inhibit phospholipase A2 activity." J Lab Clin Med, 1992: 67–77.

[109] Scott CA, Bewley S, Rudd A, Spark P, Kurinczuk JJ, Brocklehurst P, Knight M. "Incidence, risk factors, management, and outcomes of stroke in pregnancy." Obstet Gynecol 120, no. 2 Pt 1 (2012): 318-24.

[110] Sebire NJ, Fox H, Backos M, Rai R, Paterson C, Regan L. "Defective endovascular trophoblast invasion in primary antiphos- pholipid antibody syndrome-associated early pregnancy failure.." Hum Reprod, 2002: 1067–71.

[111] Shurtz-Swirski R, Inbar O, Blank M et al. "In vitro effect of anticardiolipin autoantibodies upon total and pulsatile placental hCG secretion during early pregnancy.." Am J Reprod Immunol, 1993: 206–10.

[112] Stella CL, How HY, Sibai BM. "Thrombophilia and adverse maternal-perinatal outcome: controversies in screening and management." Am J Perinatol, Nov 2006: 499-506.

[113] Sthoeger ZM, Mozes E, Tartakovsky B. "Anti-cardiolipin antibodies induce pregnancy failure by impairing embryonic implantation.." Proc Natl Acad Sci USA, 1993: 6464–646.

[114] Stirling Y, Woolf L, North WR, Seghatchian MJ, Meade TW. "Haemostasis in normal pregnancy." Thromb Haemost 52 (1984): 176 - 82

[115] Tormene D, Simioni P, Prandoni P, et al. "Factor V Leiden mutation and the risk of venous thromboembolism in pregnant women." Haematologica 86 (2001): 1305 - 1309.

[116] Vaquero E, Lazzarin N, Caserta D, Valensise H, Baldi M, Moscarini M, Arduii D. "Diagnostic evaluation of women experiencing repeated in vitro fertilization failure." Eur J Gynecol Reprod Biol 10 (2005): 1253-5.

[117] Voetsch B, Damasceno BP, Camargo EC, Massaro A, Bacheschi LA, Scaff M, Annichino-Bizzacchi JM, Arruda VR. "nherited thrombophilia as a risk factor for the development of ischemic stroke in young adults. I." Thromb Haemost 83, no. 2 (2000): 229-33.

[118] Walker JH, Boustead CM, Koster JJ, Bewley M, Waller DA. "Annexin V, a calcium-dependent phospholipid-binding protein.." Biochem Soc Trans, 1992: 828–33.

[119] Weber R, Busch E. "[Thrombophilias in patients with ischemic stroke. Indication and calculated costs for evidence-based diagnostics and treatment]." Nervenarzt 76, no. 2 (2005): 193-201.

[120] Yetman DL, Kutteh WH. "Antiphospholipid antibody panels and recurrent pregnancy loss: prevalence of anticardiolipin anti- bodies compared with other antiphospholipid antibodies." Fertil Steril, 1996: 540–546.

[121] Younis JS, Brenner B, Ohel G, Tal J, Lanir N, Ben-Ami M. Activated protein C resistance and factor V Leiden mutation can be associated with first- as well as second- trimester recurrent pregnancy loss. Am J Reprod Immunol, 2000: 31 - 5.

[122] Ziporen L, Shoenfeld Y. "Anti-phospholipid syndrome: from patient's bedside to experimental animal models and back to the patient's bedside." Hematol Cell Ther, 40 1998: 175–182.

Chapter 3

Placenta Changes During Pregnancy with Thrombophilia — Influences of Low Molecular Weight Heparin Therapy

P. Ivanov and Tsv. Tsvyatkovska

Additional information is available at the end of the chapter

1. Introduction

When there is pregnancy establishment, three separate individuals are involved in the process: the fetus, the mother, and the father. Each has its own unique genetic material, and each has its own physiologic relationship to the others in the triad. In addition to the genetic heterogeneity, there is also physiologic complex bound between the mother and fetus concluded in double circulation of the placenta. Both maternal and fetal health affects the placenta circulation, and health is a combination of genetics and environment, which add further complexity to the situation.

A recent hypothesis has been given to evaluate lesions in the placenta that are or could be associated with hypoxia of either the fetus or mother part of placental circulation. The placenta is a two-part composite organ and is sustained by blood from both the mother and the fetus. Therefore, thrombophilia (inherited or acquired) in the mother, which might result in thrombosis of the spiral arterioles, could be hypothesized to have one effect on the placenta, whereas thrombophilia in the fetus would be expected to occlude the fetal vasculature with a different pattern of pathology.

2. Maternal thrombophilia and placenta pathology findings

It is known that thrombotic tendencies in the mother associated with acquired thrombophilia, such as the antiphospholipid syndrome, may result in placental pathologic findings of decreased placental weight, infarcts, increased numbers of syncytial knots, "accelerated villous maturation" and atherosis, identical to the findings associated with severe pregnancy induced hypertension [1, 2]. Because the presumed pathogenesis of the placental pathology is thrombosis of decidual arterioles, it is a logical assumption that similar changes may be seen in the presence of maternal inherited thrombophilia. The present studies are still in contradiction regarding whether the presence of inherited thrombophilia in the mother and/or fetus is associated with placental pathologic changes [3, 4, 5]. There are many variables among the investigation that attempt to determine whether there is an association between inherited mother thrombophilia and placental pathology. Studies differ in many respects, including whether the mutation status of the mother or fetus is assessed, the type of placental lesions evaluated, and the ascertainment of the subjects.

Pathologic findings which could be supposed as a result of placental ischemia are multitude but only a couple of them could be connected with disturbance due to the presence of factors leading to thrombosis development [6, 7, 8].

Lesions hypothesized to reflect maternal thrombotic disease include placentas with weight small for gestational age (<10th percentile), infarcts, and increased numbers of syncytial knots (Tenney-Parker change). The placenta's infarcts have been defined as localized area of coagulative necrosis in the placenta's parenchyma which is confirmed histologically. Increased syncytial knots, described as excessive number of villi with prominent syncytial knots; although most commonly seen with maternal vascular underperfusion, was also assessed not only in maternal but also in fetus thrombophilia.

One of the prominent investigations concerning the impact of maternal thrombophilia on placenta changes during pregnancy was performed by Rogers et al. [9]. They found statistically significant association of increased syncytial knotting and hypervascular villi with maternal FVL mutation suggesting that hypoxia of the placental vascular bed occurs more frequently in mothers with FVL mutation than those without. Rogers et al. found more than three times prevalence of syncytial knots after investigation of 105 placenta specimens from FVL positive mothers compared with 225 controls (respectively 13% versus 4% pathological findings, p=0.004). The investigation was performed over deliveries of health newborns after 35 week of gestation and was controlled for presence of placenta's pathology influence factors such as pregnancy related hypertension, preeclampsia, small-for-gestational-age infants. They also found increased number of hypervascular villi in FVL positive mothers compared with controls (10% versus 3%, p=0.018). Placentas from infants heterozygous for FVL mutation had more avascular villi than controls (OR 2.9, 95% CI 1.5–5.6, p = 0.001). This study was performed with statistical power to patients' follow up in a prospective manner and in addition, a single pathologist, blinded to the clinical data, reviewed the slides to maintain consistency of observation.

Gogia and Machin [10] found other placenta pathology connected with thrombophilia. They established that maternal floor infarction (MFI), massive perivillous fibrin deposition (MPVFD), and fetal thrombotic vasculopathy (FTV) are specific placental lesions with associations to recurrent adverse fetal outcomes and with maternal thrombophilia. Maternal floor infarction was defined as rind of fibrinoid lining the maternal surface of the placenta. Pervillous fibrin deposition was diagnosed as transmural and not involving the placental periphery only. Fetal arterial vasculopathy was confirmed when there was no evidence of cord blood flow restriction, and thrombi were identified in stem villous arteries, with downstream avascular villi floating in a patent intervillous space. In the total of 138 investigated placentas 77% of the identified thrombophilia were genetic, and 23% were acquired. Thrombophilia was identified in 40%, 23%, and 71% respectively in cases of maternal floor infarction, perivillous fibrin deposition, and fetal thrombotic vasculopathy. The most common genetic thrombophilia was protein S deficiency, found in 39% of cases followed by FVL established in 31% of cases.

Four other published series investigated maternal and fetal thrombophilia in the context of specific placental lesions, including fetal thrombotic vasculopathy, maternal floor infarction, and massive perivillous fibrin deposition. Three of these showed an association between maternal thrombophilia and placental lesions [11, 12, 13]. Ariel et al [14] found no evidence of increased prevalence of FVL, FII 20210 G>A, and MTHFR 677 C>T in fetal DNA of 19 cases with a variety of placental lesions, including occlusive large fetal vessel disease, hyalinized avascular villi, and chorangiosis. However they did not include maternal floor infarction or perivillous fibrin deposition, and the investigation was limited to the three types genetic thrombophilia.

2.1. Conclusion

In summary, there are the alterations of the placenta indicative of the presence of inherited thrombophilia in the mother, although there are papers which have come to the conclusion that there is no clear relationship between thrombophilic mutations with placental abnormalities and/or adverse pregnancy outcomes. This is also confounded by the fact that the thrombophilic mutations are not equally frequent among the races and many studies had small sample sizes.

3. Fetal thrombophilia and placenta pathology findings

Hereditary and acquired coagulation abnormalities may contribute to hypercoagulability, especially during the second and third trimester of pregnancy which places the placenta and ultimately the fetus at risk for complications. Because the placenta is an organ with two separated by specific membrane circulations, fetal in the villi and maternal between the villi, placental thrombotic complications may include those contributed by either the mother or fetus.

Placental findings that indicate maternal thrombotic or thromboembolic events include placental infarcts in which the villi are infarcted because of maternal vascular compromise. In these cases the pathology findings are necrotic villi with collapsed or empty intervillous space (maternal lakes). Fairly rarer are placental findings that suggest a thrombosis in the fetal part of placental circulation. Fetal-side thrombosis (FST) is uncommon, but could be catastrophic for fetus fate because of the related high perinatal morbidity and mortality. Evidence of FST has been documented in cases of fetus congenital stroke [15, 16], renal vein thrombosis [17, 18], and by placental lesions [19, 20]. Thereby the term FST is related not only with placental-fetal-vascular thrombosis, but also with fetal-visceral-vascular lesions. Placenta-related FST are documented by the occurrence of a couple of different histopathological findings. First, this is macroscopic or microscopic presence of thrombosis in the fetal circulation including villous vessels, chorionic plate vessels, umbilical vessels. Second, there is hemorrhagic endovasculitis (extravasated fetal RBCs) in livebirths, related with the presence of areas of occluded villous vessel with patent (open) intervillous space in the absence of any inflammatory signs of villitis [21, 22, 23]. The mentioned thrombosis in chorionic villi, chorionic plate or umbilical vessel has been reported in 4% to 5% of all placentas examined by histology [20]. So the relation between clinical appearance and pathology finding is frequently obscure. Additionally, some maternal disorders like diabetes mellitus, and placental abnormalities such as cord anomalies, velamentous vessels, chorioamnionitis with vascular inflammation ("funisitis" or chorionic plate "vasculitis"), and multigestation are associated with placental FST. However, these associations are exceptional and the above mentioned pregnancy complications have been related mainly with maternal side placental thrombosis [24, 25].

Frequently, most placental FST present in placentas with no other findings and in patients (mothers and infants) with no known risk factors. The clinical significance of placental FST is controversial. Some authorities regarding even a single thrombus is significant [19], whereas others attach no significance to a small isolated lesion [25]. The possible association of placental FST with severe fetal conditions such as cerebral palsy or fetal/infant visceral thrombosis [26] probably warrants clinical vigilance, but in the cases of absence of specific causes targeted follow-up is difficult.

One potential cause of placental FST are hereditary haemostatic aberrations. This finding suggests that the placenta may be the cause of placental vascular insufficiencies either from maternal or fetal side complications, as suggested by some authors [27, 28]. Recently, perinatal morbidity has been studied in relation to placental FST and the potential contribution of inherited hypercoagulability in the fetus is noted as an important differential diagnosis [13]. In these cases an examination of fetus carrier status for thrombophilic mutation has been considered.

A short prospective and extended retrospective investigation connected with fetal thrombophilia and fetal-side placental thrombosis has been performed by Vern et al [12]. They evaluated 148 placentas for FST and along with this a carrier status of the fetuses for FVL and FII 20210 G>A have been performed. FST was found only in 3% of investigated placentas. One heterozygous fetus for FVL and another for FII 20210 G>A were found giving very low mutation incidences (less than 1%, in disagreement with reported 3 to 5% appearance in health Caucasian population). Because of these results, the authors proceeded to analyze a larger number of placental FST in a separate retrospective study: Five of 27 study cases (18.5%) of placental FST were identified as FVL heterozygotes by this assay. One case of heterozygosity for FVL was found among 21 control placenta cases without FTS. The numbers were small, however, compared with both sets of controls, the number of FVL in infants with placental FST was significantly increased (P <0.01). None of the known risk factors for placental FST were present in the FVL heterozygous cases: none had acute chorioamnionitis, maternal diabetes mellitus, suffered a cord accident, nor had membranous insertions of the cord. This excluded confounding factors which could be related with FST pathology. The apparent increase in the incidence of FVL in placentas with placental FST suggests that in some cases the cause of placental FST may be fetal thrombophilia. This is supported by the fact that in these identified FVL heterozygotes, none had any other known risk factor for developing placental FST. It should be noted that the mentioned study included only fetuses and placentas from normal pregnancies ended with live born fetus after 37 week of gestation. The histopathology of placenta of FVL positive stillbirth has not been discussed in this study. Because individuals with FVL carry a distinct increased risk for thrombotic complications, the authors suggest that infants (and potentially the parents of these infants), born of pregnancies complicated by FST in the placenta, should screened for FVL.

Ariel et al [14] investigated the histology findings in positive and negative FVL fetuses which were born after pregnancy with placental abruption, intrauterine growth restriction or preeclampsia. They have not found association between FVL and placental thrombotic changes, nevertheless there were 19 from 64 newborn with FVL thrombophilia (29.7%).

Other authors [29] investigated carrier status for FVL in abortive materials of pregnancies ended in first and second trimester. Along with mutation establishment, the authors examined placentas for presence of infarcts on fetal placenta side. The placental infarctions on fetal side were defined as histology findings of occluded fetal stem artery associated with infarction of the terminal villi in the distribution of the occluded vessel. So, the maternal side infarction connected with heavy deposition of fibrin in the decidua beneath the placenta rather than arterial occlusion and ischemic necrosis of the villi have been excluded. The authors found greater than twice the carrier frequency of FVL mutation in spontaneously aborted fetuses (8.6%) than in the control group (4.2%), p = 0.046. Placentas with more than 10% surface occupied by fetal side infarction were found in 42% of FVL positive fetuses compared with only 1.9% in placentas from non FVL fetuses (p<0.0001).The results suggest that FVL mutation predisposes to spontaneous miscarriage and placental infarction in cases of fetal thrombophilia.

Von Kries at al. [30] perform study over 375 Caucasian children born after 37 week of gestation pregnancy with birth weight "in the lowest quartile" for respective week of gestation. They investigated children carrier status for FVL, FII 20210 G>A, protein C, S, antithrombin III deficiency. The authors found non-significant correlation (OR 1.53 95% CI 0.76-3.08) between single mutation carrier status and significant correlation (OR 4.01 95% CI 1.48-10.84) between two or more mutation carrier status and intrauterine grow retardation (IUGR). Proportion of IUGR among children with one and two mutations was respectively 27.3% and 40%. So the authors concluded that fetal thrombophilia could be an additional cause of low birth weight.

Although it is difficult to gauge whether the presence of FVL or FII 20210 G>A may affect coagulation in the fetus, especially because fetal and neonatal levels of coagulation proteins are low and clotting indices such as prothrombin time are prolonged in comparison with adults [31], the presence of FST in placentas from pregnancies without other thrombotic risk factors strongly suggests that fetal hypercoagulopathy may exist. Concerning future treatment of FST or arranging actions against repeated incidences of FST in further pregnancy not very much could be done. As it has been known to date, the low molecular height heparins did not cross placenta so the predictable anticoagulant effect in fetus coagulation could not expected.

4. Doppler ultrasound markers and thrombophilia presence. Influence of antithrombotic therapy on uterine and placental blood flow

4.1. Introduction

The association between pregnancy complications and high incidence of acquired and congenital thrombophilia may indicate that disturbances in hemostasis lead to a prothrombotic state and may predispose affected individuals to either poor embryonic implantation in the endometrium or, later in pregnancy, to decreased placental perfusion. The proposed underlying mechanisms [32] include interference with trophoblast differentiation, inadequate placentation, or thrombosis of the placental vasculature, with consequent reduced placental perfusion, oxidative stress, and maternal endothelial dysfunction that is believed to trigger the hallmark biological and clinical manifestations of preeclampsia, IUGR or pregnancy loss.

Acquired thrombophilia such as antiphospholipid antibody syndrome has been shown to be associated with adverse pregnancy outcomes. Direct damage of trophoblast cells and utero-placental thrombosis appear to lead to the fetal manifestations of poor growth, oligohydramnios and abnormal Doppler velocimetry. There is some evidence in antiphospholipid antibody syndrome that treatment with heparin corrects the abnormality in trophoblast invasion and thrombosis, and also decreases the fetal loss rate. Numerous conflicting studies suggest a relationship between adverse pregnancy outcomes and genetic thrombophilia. The pathogenesis of the disease is likely to be very similar to antiphospholipid antibody syndrome though data is limited. But there are considerable controversies about the influence of genetic thrombophilia on the ultrasound markers associated with blood flow in the uterine arteries, circulation in placental vessels and umbilical cord.

Failure of trophoblastic invasion has been found to be associated with uteroplacental insufficiency. Doppler measured parameters both in first and second trimesters have demonstrated an association between the increased impedance of flow in the uterine arteries and subsequent development of preeclampsia, IUGR, and fetal death. Doppler ultrasound predicts the development of severe preeclampsia with higher sensitivity and specificity, compared with pregnancy-induced hypertension. For example Papageorghiou et al [33] demonstrated that increased pulsatility index (PI) on Doppler ultrasound was identified in 41% of women who later developed preeclampsia. The sensitivities for preeclampsia requiring delivery before 36, 34, and 32 weeks were 70%, 81%, and 90%, respectively. Doppler ultrasound has also been used in the first trimester to predict preeclampsia. The likelihood ratio (LR) for the development of PE was about 5 and for those with normal Doppler results the LR was about 0.5 [34]. Similarly, the LR of developing IUGR is about 4 in women with evidence of increased impedance of blood flow on Doppler. The main preventive approach in this approach to escape this pregnancy complication has been connected with low molecular weight heparin application. LMWHs with long half-lives, resulting in the need for less frequent injections, have made them attractive for practical use during the 9 months of pregnancy. In addition, the widespread use over the last 10 years has shown that LMWHs are safer than unfractionated heparin (UH) during pregnancy. Many studies have indicated that LMWHs are one of the factors regulating trophoblast invasion, although the results were not always consistent. In 2006, Erden et al. [35] found the underlying mechanism involved in the improvement of trophoblast invasion using LMWH in patients with a history of miscarriage. They reported that enoxaparin can reduce E-cadherin expression but not laminin expression in rat pregnancy, which might modulate trophoblast invasion. The antithrombotic action and the amelioration of blood flow rheology of LMWH in developed intervillous space in second trimester of pregnancy are believed to improve Doppler sonographic markers. The discovery of discreet Doppler alterations in placental and uterine artery blood flow could help in early steps of pregnancy rescue.

4.2. Doppler ultrasound markers and thrombophilia presence

One of the first authors who investigated connection between thrombophilia and impaired blood flow during pregnancy were Grandone et al. [36] They found persistent in second trimester of pregnancy bilateral uterine artery notches during Doppler blood flow examination in 41 women with inherited thrombophilia (FVL, FII 20210 G>A, antithrombin III, protein C or protein S deficiency). This finding is associated with six-fold higher risk of having an adverse outcome compared with women without these thrombophilic conditions.

Other studies again evaluated the presence of an association between common prothrombotic factors and increased blood flow resistance in the fetomaternal circulation, connected with obstetric complications occurrence. The investigators [37] did not find an association between thrombophilia and blood flow in the fetomaternal circulation in nulliparous women.

Useful information was found in Doppler sound characteristics investigation of uterine artery flow in non-pregnant women with recurrent pregnancy loss history. Lazzarine et al [38] investigated PI values of uterine artery in midluteal phase of 230 women who had experienced two or more first trimester pregnancy loss (RPL). Uterine arteries PI values in RPL patients (2.42 ±0.79) were significantly higher with respect to those found in the control group (2.08 ± 0.47). When patients were grouped according to the different RSA causes, the highest PI values were found among patients with uterine abnormalities (2.82 ± 1.0), antiphospholipid antibodies syndrome (2.70 ± 1.1), and unexplained RSA (2.60 ± 0.7). These values were significantly higher with respect to that found in the control group. No differences were observed in PI values between fertile patients and those with RSA due to thyroid abnormalities (2.10 ± 0.55), inherited thrombophilia (2.03 ± 0.45), autoimmune pathology (2.34 ±1.18), and genetic anomalies (2.47 ± 0.54). Similar results were observed when patients were grouped according to primary and secondary RPL. According to the results, the increased resistance of uterine blood flow in non-pregnant uterus may be an important sign to some causes of RPL and may represent an independent indication of careful further pregnancy follow up.

When talking about fetus thrombophilic status, there should be mentioned the important influence of non-mother thrombophilic conditions and the disturbance of umbilical blood flow. Lindqvist et al [39] investigated umbilical artery Doppler velocimetry on 54 women in late pregnancy. They found that abnormal umbilical artery Doppler velocimetry was associated with an approximately seven-fold increased risk of fetoplacental thrombotic vasculopathy (OR: 7.5, 95% CI: 1.3-44.3), ischemic lesions (OR: 7.5, 95% CI: 1.2-46.1) and fetal carriership of FVL (OR: 8.2, 95% CI: 1.5-43.5). The study gives power of FVL-fetus carriership and pregnancy complications connected with fetal demise.

4.3. Influence of antithrombotic therapy on uterine and placental blood flow

In the follow up of women with inherited and acquired thrombophilia using LMWH Cok et al [40] did not find significant positive influence of the therapy with heparins on the uterine artery blood flow. They concluded that the administration of LMWH (enoxaparine 40 mg daily) throughout the pregnancy in patients with thrombophilia does not prevent the increase of uterine artery Doppler flow indices and IUGR, which is probably as a result of defective trophoblastic invasion. Investigation of Doppler parameters was performed during the 18–22-week period of gestation over 64 pregnant women who experienced minimum three previous pregnancy loss after ten weeks of gestation and who had acquired or inherited thrombophilia (positive lupus anticoagulant, antiphospholipid antibody, FVL, FII 20210 G>A, antithrombin III, protein C or S deficiency). The authors found increased impedance to blood flow in the uterine arteries which is associated with increased risk for subsequent development of preeclampsia, IUGR, and perinatal death in thrombophilia presence. Despite LMWH therapy, the mean PI (1.07 ± 0.46 for LMWH group and 0.91 ± 0.31 for control, $p=0.036$) and the mean RI (0.59 ± 0.12 for LMWH group and 0.54 ± 0.10 for control, $p=0.021$) were significantly higher in the trombophilia group. These results should be interpreted with care because of relatively small investigated group and the diversity type of thrombophilia among pregnant women. Another open question is the dose regiment of LMWH therapy arranged accordingly thrombophilia type.

On the contrary, Magriples et al [41] found positive effect of anticoagulation therapy over Doppler sonographic finding in retrospective study of 51 women with inherited thrombophilia (FVL, FII 20210 G>A, MTHFR 677 C>T). In the treatment group thrombophilic women used unfractionated heparin or low molecular weight heparin for FVL and FII 20210 G>A in prophylactic doses. Heparin was used at prophylactic doses until the third trimester. In the third trimester, patients were advanced to therapeutic doses of heparin and switched to unfractionated heparin at 36 weeks. From the total of 178 monitored pregnancies, the authors reported abnormal ultrasounds significantly greater in the untreated compared with the treated with heparins pregnancies (52.8% versus 27.9%, p=0.024). Growth restrictions were more common in untreated pregnancies. There was a significantly decreased risk of oligohydramnios with treatment (27.3% versus 7%, p=0.03). Overall outcomes were significantly improved with the use of anticoagulation (p<0.0001). In a part of the cases despite treatment, oligohydramnios and growth disturbances still occurred. As heparin does not cross the fetal side of the placenta, this may account for the persistence of the poor outcomes because of positive fetus thrombophilia phenotype. The study markedly established the connection between ultrasound parameters finding for growth, fluid and feto-placental blood flow in patients with pregnant thrombophilic women and the application of anticoagulant therapy.

In a small observational study Alkazaleh et al [42] also found beneficial effect of LMWH therapy over Doppler placental flow and fetal outcome in women with previous history with pregnancy complications. They also draw attention over earlier application of LMWH therapy in indicated cases (not later than 18 to 20 week of gestation). This opens the question for window of Doppler sonographic screening and well-timed therapeutic intervention in high risk pregnancy.

4.4. Conclusion

Giving the cost and potential side effects of heparins during pregnancy, the deployment of a strategy of placental function screening using Doppler ultrasound and adding antithrombotic therapy only in the accurate cases is an appropriate clinical strategy. LMWH's therapy should be reserved for high risk populations with inherited thrombophilia mutations (double mutation carriers or thromboembolic incidences history). In non-pregnant women the Doppler examination of the uterine artery represents a useful tool for screening women with a history of RPL and, therefore, should be included in the RPL diagnostic flow chart. This test provides the opportunity to identify women in whom appropriate therapeutic protocols may effectively improve the possibility for a successfully pregnancy.

5. General conclusions

The authors who found correlation between placenta pathological findings and thrombophilia strongly advocate thrombophilia testing in all cases in which the placenta shows signs of chronic ischemic disturbance. They also recommend a full-pedigree work up including fetal and father thrombophilia screening. This approach is coming from possible multigenic effect over placenta structure coming from both maternal and fetal genotype.

The results as a whole suggest that these unusual forms of fibrin deposition (not thrombosis), increased numbers of syncytial knots and maternal side placental infarcts are frequently associated with thrombophilia. In a part of cases – in maternal floor infarction there is 50% recurrence rate suggests an interaction between maternal and fetal thrombophilia, resulting in a "plane of fibrin deposition" in which the maternal and fetal circulations overlap across the entire placental bed. Only about in 40% of cases of placentas with histopathology showing chronic ischemia have identifiable thrombophilia. The reasons for this may include other thrombophilia not discovered or not investigated in the give study or presences of other (mechanical?) factors impede blood flow in the intervillous space.

Author details

P. Ivanov[1,2] and Tsv. Tsvyatkovska[2]

1 Clinical Institute for Reproductive Medicine, Pleven, Bulgaria

2 Department of Biochemistry, Medical University of Pleven, Bulgaria

References

[1] Levy, R. A, Avvad, E, Oliveira, J, & Porto, L. C. Placental pathology in antiphospholipid syndrome. Lupus. (1998). SS85., 81.

[2] Abramowsky, C. R, Vegas, M. E, Swinehart, G, & Gyves, M. T. Decidual vasculopathy of the placenta in lupus erythematosus. NEJM. (1980). , 303, 668-672.

[3] Redline, R. W. Thrombophilia and placental pathology. Clin Obstet Gynecol. (2006). , 49, 885-894.

[4] Katz, V. L. Di Tomasso J, Farmer R, Carpenter M. Activated protein C resistance associated with maternal floor infarction treated with low-molecular-weight heparin. Am J Perinatol. (2002). , 19, 273-277.

[5] Many, A, Schreiber, L, Rosner, S, Lessing, J. B, Eldor, A, & Kupferminc, M. J. Pathologic features of the placenta in women with severe pregnancy complications and thrombophilia. Obstet Gynecol. (2001). , 98, 1041-1044.

[6] Kraus, F. T, Redline, R. W, Gersell, D. J, Nelson, D. M, & Dicke, J. M. editors. of the Atlas of Nontumor Pathology. 2. Armed Forces Institute of Pathology; Washington, DC: American Registry of Pathology; (2004). Placental Pathology., 3

[7] Redline, R. W, Boyd, T, Campbell, V, Hyde, S, Kaplan, C, Khong, T. Y, Prashner, H. R, & Waters, B. L. Maternal vascular underperfusion: nosology and reproducibility of placental reaction patterns. Pediatr Dev Pathol. (2004). , 7, 237-249.

[8] Redline, R. W, Ariel, I, Baergen, R. N, Desa, D. J, Kraus, F. T, Roberts, D. J, & Sander, C. M. Fetal vascular obstructive lesions: nosology and reproducibility of placental reaction patterns. Pediatr Dev Pathol. (2004). , 7, 443-452.

[9] Rogers, B. B, Momirova, V, Dizon-townson, D, Wenstrom, K, Samuels, P, Sibai, B, Spong, C, Caritis, S. N, Sorokin, Y, Miodovnik, M, Sullivan, O, Conway, M. J, & Wapner, D. RJ. Avascular villi, increased syncytial knots, and hypervascular villi are associated with pregnancies complicated by factor V Leiden mutation. Pediatr Dev Pathol. (2010). , 13, 341-7.

[10] Gogia, N, & Machin, G. A. Maternal thrombophilias are associated with specific placental lesions. Pediatr Dev Pathol. (2008). , 11, 424-9.

[11] Arias, F, Romero, R, Joist, H, & Kraus, F. T. Thrombophilia: a mechanism of disease in women with adverse pregnancy outcome and thrombotic lesions in the placenta. J Matern-Fetal Med (1998). , 7, 277-286.

[12] Vern, T. Z, Alles, A. J, Kowal-vern, A, Longtine, J, & Roberts, D. J. Frequency of Factor V Leiden and prothrombin G20210A in placentas and their relationship with placental lesions. Hum Pathol (2000). , 31, 1036-1043.

[13] Kraus, F, & Acheen, V. I. Fetal thrombotic vasculopathy in the placenta: cerebral thrombi and infarcts, coagulopathies, and cerebral palsy. Hum Pathol (1999). , 30, 759-769.

[14] Ariel, I, Anteby, E, Hamani, Y, & Redline, R. W. Placental pathology in fetal thrombophilia. Hum Pathol (2004). , 35, 729-733.

[15] Silver, R. K. MacGregor SN, Pasternak JF, et al: Fetal stroke associated with elevated maternal anticardiolipin antibodies. Obstet Gynecol (1992). , 80, 497-499.

[16] Koelfen, W, & Freund, M. Varnholt V: Neonatal stroke involving the middle cerebral artery in term infants: Clinical presentation, EEG and imaging studies, and outcome. Dev Med Child Neurol (1995). , 37, 204-212.

[17] Oppenheimer, E. H. Esterly JR: Thrombosis in a newborn: comparison between infants of diabetic and nondiabetic mothers. J Pediatr (1965). , 67, 549-556.

[18] Alexander, F. Campbell WAB: Congenital nephrotic syndrome and renal vein thrombosis in infancy. J Clin Pathol (1971). , 24, 27-40.

[19] Kraus FT: Placental thrombi and related problemsSemin Diagn Path (1993). , 10, 275-283.

[20] Redline, R. W. Pappin A: Fetal thrombotic vasculopathy: The clinical significance of extensive avascular villi. Hum Pathol (1995). , 26, 80-85.

[21] Sander CM: Update: Etiologydiagnosis and management of hemorrhagic endovasculitis of the placenta. Compr Ther (1991). , 17, 16-19.

[22] Salafia, C. M, Pezzullo, J. C, Minior, V. K, et al. Placental pathology of absent and reversed end-diastolic flow in growth-restricted fetuses. Obstet Gynecol (1997). , 90, 830-836.

[23] Altemani, A. M. Sarian MZ: Hemorrhagic endovasculitis of the placenta: A clinical-pathological study in Brazil. J Perinat Med (1995). , 23, 359-363.

[24] Benirschke, K. Kaufman P: The Pathology of the Human Placenta (ed 3). New York, NY, Springer-Verlag, (1995). , 357-366.

[25] Fox H: Pathology of the Placenta (ed 2)Major Problems in Pathology, London, United Kingdom, Saunders, (1997). , 7, 118-122.

[26] Redline, R. W, Wilson-costello, D, Borawski, E, et al. Placental lesions associated with neurologic impairment and cerebral palsy in very low-birth-weight infants. Arch Pathol Lab Med (1998). , 122, 1091-1098.

[27] Rai, R, Regan, L, Hadley, E, et al. Second-trimester pregnancy loss is associated with activated C resistance. Br J Haematol (1996). , 92, 489-490.

[28] Rai RlRegan L, Chitolie A, et al: Placental thrombosis and second trimester miscarriage in association with activated protein C resistance. Br J Obstet Gynaecol (1996). , 103, 842-844.

[29] Dizon-townson, D. S, Meline, L, Nelson, L. M, Varner, M, & Ward, K. Fetal carriers of the factor V Leiden mutation are prone to miscarriage and placental infarction. Am J Obstet Gynecol (1997). , 177, 402-405.

[30] Von Kries, R, Junker, R, Oberle, D, Kosch, A, & Nowak-göttl, U. Foetal growth restriction in children with prothrombotic risk factors. Thromb Haemost (2001). , 86, 1012-1016.

[31] Reverdiau-moalic, P, Delahousse, B, Body, G, et al. Evolution of blood coagulation activators and inhibitors in the healthy human fetus. Blood (1996). , 88, 900-906.

[32] Kahn, S. R, Platt, R, Mcnamara, H, Rozen, R, & Chen, M. F. Genest J Jr, Goulet L, Lydon J, Seguin L, Dassa C, Masse A, Asselin G, Benjamin A, Miner L, Ghanem A, Kramer MS ((2009). Inherited thrombophilia and preeclampsia within a multicenter cohort: the Montreal Preeclampsia Study. Am J Obstet Gynecol 2009; 200:151.e, 1-9.

[33] Papageorghiou, A. T, & Yu, C. K. Nicolaides KH: The role of uterine artery Doppler in predicting adverse pregnancy outcome. Best Pract Res Clin Obstet Gynaecol (2004). , 18, 383-396.

[34] Nicolaides, K. H, Bindra, R, Turan, O. M, et al. A novel approach to first-trimester screening for early pre-eclampsia combining serum and Doppler ultrasound. Ultrasound Obstet Gynecol (2006). , 13.

[35] Erden, O, Imir, A, Guvenal, T, Muslehiddinoglu, A, Arici, S, Cetin, M, & Cetin, A. Investigation of the effects of heparin and low molecular- weight heparin on E-cadherin and laminin expression in rat pregnancy by immunohistochemistry. Hum Reprod (2006). , 21, 3014-3018.

[36] Grandone, E, Colaizzo, D, Martinelli, P, & Paladini, D. di Minno G, Margaglione M. Adverse outcome in women with thrombophilia and bilateral uterine artery notches. Fertil Steril (2006). , 86, 726-727.

[37] Salomon, O, Seligsohn, U, Steinberg, D. M, Zalel, Y, Lerner, A, Rosenberg, N, Pshithizki, M, et al. The common prothrombotic factors in nulliparous women do not compromise blood flow in the fetomaternal circulation and are not associated with preeclampsia or intrauterine growth restriction. Am J Obstet Gynecol (2004). , 191, 2002-2009.

[38] Lazzarin, N, Vaquero, E, Exacoustos, C, Romanini, E, Amadio, A, & Arduini, D. Midluteal phase Doppler assessment of uterine artery blood flow in nonpregnant women having a history of recurrent spontaneous abortions: correlation to different etiologies. Fertil Steril (2007). , 87, 1383-1387.

[39] Lindqvist, P. G, Procházka, M, Laurini, R, & Maršál, K. Umbilical artery Doppler in relation to placental pathology and FV Leiden in pregnant women and their offspring. J Matern Fetal Neonatal Med. (2013). under press]

[40] Cok, T, Tarim, E, & Iskender, C. Comparison of uterine artery Doppler in pregnant women with thrombophilia treated by LMWHs and without thrombophilia. Arch Gynecol Obstet. (2012). , 286, 575-579.

[41] Magriples, U, Ozcan, T, Karne, A, & Copel, J. A. The effect of anticoagulation on antenatal ultrasound findings in pregnant women with thrombophilia. J Matern Fetal Neonatal Med. (2006). , 19, 27-30.

[42] Alkazaleh, F, Viero, S, Simchen, M, Walker, M, Smith, G, Laskin, C, Windrim, R, & Kingdom, J. Ultrasound diagnosis of severe thrombotic placental damage in the second trimester: an observational study. Ultrasound Obstet Gynecol. (2004). , 23, 472-6.

Chapter 4

Pharmacogenetics and the Treatment of Thrombophilia

Ivana Novaković, Nela Maksimović and Dragana Cvetković

Additional information is available at the end of the chapter

1. Introduction

Inherited forms of thrombophilia such as factor V Leiden mutation (FVL), prothrombin gene mutation (PT 20210A), and deficiencies of natural anticoagulants protein C, protein S, and antithrombin are well known. DNA tests for factor V Leiden and PT 20210A mutation have been incorporated in clinical practice for several years [1,2,3]. A number of studies have analyzed how this and other molecular genetic testing alter the clinical management and treatment of patients with thromboembolic disease or pregnancy complications. Data regarding the influence of the genotype to the disease phenotype as well as pharmacogenetic data are still controversial and emerging.

Several topics are of particular interest. Usually genetic tests follow standard investigation of coagulation cascade, but some laboratories perform them in initially. Testing of first-degree relatives of a diagnosed carrier of a thrombophilic trait is still not consecutive. Administration of anticoagulant therapy is followed by genetic tests also; DNA variations are associated with variations in drug efficacy and toxicity, particularly in cases of warfarin and clopidogrel. Investigation of inherited thrombophilia and its treatment in women with reproductive challenges, including *in vitro* fertilization (IVF), is another important question. Finally, recommendation for genetic testing and treatment of thrombophilia in children, as vulnerable group, should be clarified.

2. Thromophilia screening and treatment in asymptomatic adult carriers

Thrombophilia testing is one of the most common genetic tests ordered by clinicians [4]. Current guidelines recommend screening for inherited thrombophilia only in selected group of patients with venous thromboembolism, dependently of the age of onset, the circumstances of thrombosis, and the severity of the clinical manifestations [5,6].

When the results of the index patients are positive asymptomatic relatives often come with requests for thrombophilia testing. To date, there is variety of published guidelines. However, the utility of family testing remains matter of debate and it should be done with caution. It is a general knowledge that genetic testing is justified only if the results are likely to change medical management. American College of Medical Genetics (ACMG) and Evaluation of Genomic Applications in Practice and Prevention (EGAPP) working group published consensus statements on FVL and FII. According to ACMG it is not recommended to perform random screening of general population or prenatal and routine newborn screening [7]. Based on the current knowledge, identification of thrombophilic disorders in asymptomatic individuals would not lead to long-term treatment with anticoagulants since the risk of bleeding is higher than the risk of venous thromboembolism (VTE) [7]. The overall annual incidence of the first VTE in individuals with antithrombin, protein C or protein S deficiency is ~1.5 %, whereas for the factor V Leiden or prothrombin 20210A mutation heterozygote this risk is ~0.5% [8]. Annual major bleeding risk associated with continuous anticoagulant treatment is around 2% and it overweighs the risk of VTE [9]. The results of Middeldorp et al. on asymptomatic carriers of FVL, are in agreement with the above and since there is no clear evidence of the benefit of thrombophylaxis they do not recommend routine screening of families of symptomatic patients [10]. Also, Coppens et al. do not recommend testing first degree relatives of probands with the prothrombin 20210A mutation based on the results of a large prospective cohort study in which the annual incidence of a first VTE in PT carriers was 0.37% [11]. For asymptomatic family members who are homozygous for FVL mutation the risk increases to closely 2%. According to EGAPP the risk is sufficient to consider anticoagulation therapy but there are still no data about the outcomes [12].

The practice of family testing has been most useful for women from thrombophilic families who intend to be pregnant. Affected female relatives with antithrombin, protein C and protein S deficiency as well as FVL and 20210A mutation carriers have VTE incidence as high as 4% per pregnancy while women homozygous for FVL have the risk of 16% per pregnancy in the absence of prophylaxis [13]. In these cases anticoagulant therapy, usually low molecular heparin injections, is frequently applied.

Genetic testing is also very useful for women from thrombophilic families who wish to use oral contraceptives. Use of oral contraceptives increases the risk of VTE for women with antithrombin, protein C or protein S protein deficiency or FVL and 20210A mutation. However, it is important to know that women from thrombophilic families are at the increased risk (compared with the general population) even if they do not have these specific deficiencies or mutations, due to the other cosegregating thrombophilic defects [8]. Thus, a negative thrombophilia test may give them false reassurance.

Family testing may also help reduce VTE risk for women who tested positive through avoidance of postmenopausal hormone therapy. Advantages of testing are even higher for women considering postmenopausal hormone therapy than oral contraceptives, due to the much higher absolute risk of VTE in middle-aged than in younger women [13].

3. Antithrombotic therapy and the promise of pharmacogenetics

The expansion of pharmacogenetics, the study of genetic variants relevant to variations in drug efficacy and toxicity, and pharmacogenomics, referred to as a whole-genome application of pharmacogenetics, allowed rapid progress towards the goal of personalized therapy, tailored for individual patients [14-17].

The research in this field provides large amounts of individual-specific information concerning risk for adverse reactions or lack of drug efficacy, thus it could have significant influence on clinical practice. The question of how to use the pharmacogenetic information to improve health outcomes gains continuously increasing attention [18-20]. Specifically, it has been shown that pharmacogenetic information has the potential to improve the efficacy and safety of major antithrombotic drugs (e.g. [21]).

3.1. Warfarin: A case in point

One of the most compelling examples of potential benefits from pharmacogenomic testing is warfarin [22]. Warfarin is a widely prescribed oral anticoagulant; for decades it has been used as standard drug to prevent and treat thrombotic events in patients with deep vein thrombosis, various hypercoagulable states, atrial fibrillation, surgical cardiac valve replacement, etc.

One of the major problems with its use in clinical practice is large interindividual variation – patients differ in sensitivity to warfarin, hence the dose requirements vary widely (up to 20-fold) [19,23]. The consequences of over- or under-anticoagulation can be serious. In patients less sensitive than typical, the standard doses may be too low to achieve anticoagulation and therapeutic failure may occur, while in highly sensitive individuals the same doses may lead to serious adverse effects, such as hemorrhage.

Numerous factors are known to impact dose variation, including age, dietary vitamin K intake, presence of other comorbidities and interactions with other drugs, as well as genetic variants. The identification of these variants, and the potential use of pharmacogenetic testing to predict the appropriate drug dosing have attracted much research interest [23-28].

Prior work pointed to significant genetic component underlying variations in warfarin sensitivity. Pharmacogenetic studies identified polymorphisms in genes *CYP2C9* and *VKORC1* as principal genetic determinants of warfarin dose [23,24,29].

CYP2C9 gene encodes one of the major cytochrome P450 drug-metabolizing enzymes; it is involved in metabolic clearance of S-warfarin, the more potent isomer of warfarin, which is largely responsible for its therapeutic effects. Two common alleles are described, *CYP2C9*2* and *CYP2C9*3*, based on non-synonymous SNPs that result in Arg144Cys (*2) and Ile358Leu (*3) substitutions; both variants are associated with reduced metabolic clearance of S-warfarin, thus lowering dose requirements [24]. Carriers of these variants show high sensitivity to drug and increased risk for hemorrhagic complications compared to individuals homozygous for allele *1. It is estimated that SNPs in *CYP2C9* gene account for approximately 12% of the total variance in required warfarin dose [23] (range 6–18%, [18]).

Larger proportion of the dose variance, up to 30%, is explained by SNPs in the gene *VKORC1* [25,29]. *VKORC1* encodes vitamin K epoxide reductase complex, the target enzyme inhibited by warfarin; this enzyme is necessary for the recycling of vitamin K and consequently for activation of several clotting factors. Currently, several *VKORC1* SNPs are described (the major one being *VKORC1* -1639G>A, a common polymorphism of the promoter sequence) that define two common haplotypes, A and B. Haplotype A is associated with higher warfarin sensitivity, and hence lower mean drug doses required, contrary to B haplotype [29].

With respect to frequencies of these variants, genetic differences between populations are also a matter of great interest. The common *CYP2C9* alleles *2 and *3, associated with high warfarin sensitivity, are present in approximately 30% of people of European descent (range 13-35%), but are less frequent in those of Asian (1-12%) and African descent (0-12%) [21,25,30]. *VKORC1* B haplotype, associated with low warfarin sensitivity, is more common in European and African populations, while 'high sensitivity' A haplotype predominates in Asian populations. The frequency of A is reported as 75–92% in Asians, compared to approximately 40% in Europeans or 9–12% in people of African descent [21].

To predict response to treatment, considering polymorphisms in both genes simultaneously is of great importance. Carriers of variants associated with 'high sensitivity' at both loci are at much higher risk of over-anticoagulation [31]. On the other hand, individuals who are *CYP2C9*1*1-VKORC1*BB show less warfarin sensitivity and require higher drug dose for therapeutic anticoagulation [25]. The associated variants in both genes are thought to account for approximately 45% of response variance in European and 30% in African populations [21].

The frequency of *VKORC1* and *CYP2C9* alleles was also investigated in Serbian population, among patients under oral anticoagulant therapy [32,33]. In a group of patients with extremely unstable anticoagulant response, 89.7% were carriers of 'sensitivity' alleles, and 25% carried these variants at both *CYP2C9* and *VKORC1* loci [33].

A recent genome wide association study (GWAS) by Takeuchi et al. confirmed polymorphisms in genes *VKORC1* and *CYP2C9* as principal genetic determinants of warfarin dose and also found weaker, but still significant effect of polymorphism in another CYP gene, *CYP4F2* [23]. The effect of *CYP4F2* rs2108622 was confirmed by other authors (e.g. [26,34]).

The results concerning possible contribution of other candidate genes are still inconsistent. The investigation of other SNPs and CNVs (copy number variations) did not reveal new significant warfarin associations [23], however, limited positive data was obtained for polymorphisms in additional candidate genes such as *POR* (encoding cytochrome P450 oxidoreductase) or *CALU* (encoding calumenin) (review in [27]).

The additional polymorphisms in these or other genes relevant to blood coagulation may be worth further investigation, especially in non-European populations that were less studied pharmacogenetically [27,28].

4. Clinical application of pharmacogenetic testing — Promises and problems

What are the promises and problems of the genotype-guided antithrombotic therapy? Pharmacogenetic testing has the potential to improve the efficacy and safety of warfarin and other antithrombotic drugs [21].

Recognizing the significance of the genetic information, US FDA added it to warfarin label in 2007 and suggested that clinicians considered genetic testing before initiating therapy. Genetic tests for CYP2C9 and VKORC1 'sensitivity' variants are available for clinical use, and so are dosing algorithms that combine genetic and clinical data [35,36]. Including CYP4F2 rs2108622 in testing procedures and algorithms is also suggested [27].

However, the question of routine adoption of pharmacogenetic testing for warfarin sensitivity into clinical practice has led to vigorous debates. Numerous problems and challenges arise, from cost-effectiveness analyses, possibility of development of alternative drugs [27], complexity, quality and time demands, the need for additional education and training, to ethical and regulatory issues [19,21,36].

The major issue for clinical application of pharmacogenetic testing is that this approach must provide significant benefit to patients compared to nongenetic approach only. Cost-effectiveness emerges as another important question in modern health care; currently, discussions are focused on the cost of genetic testing *vs.* potential savings by reducing severe health complications [18,19,31,37]. Also, the aim is to identify specific groups of patients who will benefit most from the pharmacogenetic testing [20], and to obtain diversity of warfarin dosing algorithms that should reflect genetic diversity of populations [28].

A multicenter study, published in 2009 by the International 'Warfarin Pharmacogenetics Consortium, demonstrated that algorithms for warfarin dosing that incorporate pharmacogenomic information were better than those using clinical data alone [35]. The greatest benefits were observed in patients with extreme (very low or very high) dose requirements. A recent Medco-Mayo Warfarin Effectiveness study demonstrated that application of warfarin genotyping significantly reduced the incidence of hospitalizations due to bleeding and thromboembolism [37]. Eckman and colleagues analyzed cost-effectiveness of using pharmacogenetic approach for patients with atrial fibrillation and concluded that genotype-guided warfarin therapy might be cost effective in a high-risk group [31].

However, general consensus regarding these questions is lacking. The results of the ongoing studies and trials, conducted on large scales and diverse populations, are expected to clarify these issues [21].

With the current pace of pharmacogenetic discoveries, integrating the growing amount of individual-specific data into clinical practice to improve health outcome will remain the challenging task.

5. Genetics and treatment of reproductive adversity in thrombophilia

Clinical manifestations and morbidity associated with thrombophilia in pregnancy include pregnancy loss, as well as other adverse outcomes eg. preeclampsia, placental abruption, and intrauterine growth restriction. Pregnancy-related thromboembolism is also part of thrombophilia spectrum making the influence of thrombophilia in pregnancy is an important and interesting research topic.

The effect of preventive anticoagulant therapy during the pregnancy in women with inherited thrombophila is still controversial. Early investigations were characterized by small participant numbers, poor study design and heterogeneity. The debate on the efficacy of aspirin and heparin has advanced with recently published randomised-controlled trials. One large Italian study encompassed 1011 pregnancies of 416 women who were carriers of factor V Leiden (FVL) mutation and/or prothrombin gene variant G20210A (PTG) [38]. The outcome was evaluated according to the type of treatment (low molecular weight heparin and/or aspirin) and the period of pregnancy when the treatment started. The results showed that low molecular weight heparin (LMWH) had a protective effect on miscarriages (odds ratio, OR 0.52) and venous thromboembolism (OR 0.05) while aspirin administration showed no advantage on the prevention of obstetric complications and venous thromboembolism (OR 2.2 and 0.48, respectively). These results suggest that LMWH prophylaxis reduces the risk of obstetric complications in carriers of FVL and/or PTG, particularly in those with previous obstetric events. Mitic et al. also reported significant improvement of pregnancy outcome after implementation of thromboprophylaxis in Serbian patients with inherited thrombophilia and previous pregnancy losses [39].

One Bulgarian group reported their first experience with management of inherited thrombophilia during pregnancy [40]. After the testing for factor V Leiden, prothrombin G20210A, plasminogen activator inhibitor-1 (PAI-1) 4G/4G and PAI-1 4G/5G they established a diagnosis of inherited thrombophilia in 72% (24 out of 38) patients with history of an abnormal pregnancy (miscarriage, still birth, placental abruption, preeclampsia and intrauterine fetal growth restriction). All diagnosed patients were treated with aspirin (75mg) prior to conception and low molecular heparin after detection of fetal heart sounds. Anticoagulant treatment of these patients was deemed successful with 87.5% (21 out of 24) giving birth to a term newborn.

However, several investigators have reported confounding experiences [41-43]. In a recently published review, de Jong et al suggest that the association between inherited thrombophilia and recurrent miscarriage is not very strong, and the evidence does not indicate that the use of anticoagulants improves the chance of live birth in these women [41]. The authors conclude that by the current state of evidence, testing for inherited thrombophilia should not lead to altered clinical management and so, should not be performed routinely in women with recurrent miscarriage. In light of the available data, a well-designed, multi-center collaboration is required to ascertain the effect of inherited thrombophilia on early pregnancy loss and to establish evidence-based treatment recommendations [44].

It may be possible that in women with recurrent pregnancy loss multiple thrombophilic gene mutations rather than specific single gene changes play a role. In one study, 10 gene mutations were analyzed: factor V Leiden, factor V H1299R (R2), factor V Y1702C, prothrombin gene G20210A, factor XIII V34L, beta-fibrinogen -455G>A, PAI-1 4G/5G, human platelet alloantigen a/b (L33P), methylenetetrahydrofolate reductase C677T and A1298C [45]. There were no differences in the frequency of specific mutations in women with recurrent miscarriage compared to healthy control. However, the prevalence of homozygous mutations and total gene mutations was significantly higher in patients compared to controls. Homozygous mutations were found in 59% of women with a history of recurrent pregnancy loss vs. 10% of control women. More than three gene mutations were observed in 68% of women with recurrent miscarriage compared to 21% of controls. It would be of especial interest to explore how number of detected mutations influences effects of prophylactic therapy and further reproductive outcome.

The possible connection between inherited thrombophilia and outcomes of *in vitro* fertilization (IVF) is another challenging topic. A number of investigations suggest no association of thrombophilic mutations and IVF pregnancy failure [46,47]. Rudick et al. found a very low prevalence of FVL mutation in women in their IVF program (1.6%), and suggested a positive association between this genetic marker and pregnancy [47]. The authors suggested that routine testing in a general IVF population for FVL mutation as a cause of IVF failure and infertility is not indicated. Ricci et al. compared the prevalence of FVL and PTG mutation in women undergoing IVF to women with spontaneous pregnancy, as well as IVF outcomes and the risk of complications in FVL and PTG carriers to non-carriers [48]. In this prospective cohort study they found the same prevalence of thrombophilic mutations in women requiring IVF and in women with spontaneous pregnancy. The results of this study also suggested the presence of FVL and PTG in asymptomatic women and in the absence of other risk factors did not influence IVF outcome, represent a risk for ovarian hyperstimulation syndrome, or favor thrombosis after IVF. According to these authors, screening for FVL and PTG does not appear to be justified to identify the patients at the risk for IVF failure or associated complications.

However, some studies have shown positive effects of LMWH treatment for women with thrombophilia and recurrent IVF- embrio transfer failures [49,50]. In one prospective randomized placebo-controlled trial Qublan et al. observed that implantation rate, pregnancy and live birth rates are significantly increased with LMWH compared to placebo [49]. At this moment, diagnostic tools to identify patients at risk of implantation failure are still limited and therapeutic options to improve implantation rates are far from being established. In addition to genetic markers of thrombophilia and thromboprophylaxis, different immunological mechanisms and consecutive immunomodulatory treatments are the subjects of intensive investigations [51].

6. Thrombophilia screening in asymptomatic children

Parents with known specific thrombophilic defect frequently ask whether or not their child(ren) should also be screened for thrombophilia. Many of them are concerned about their children's health, mostly the risk of having VTE or reproductive issues, especially if the mother was diagnosed during pregnancy or after several pregnancy losses. Genetic testing is particularly controversial in children since their decision-making capability is non-existent or is limited [52].

The recommendation of The American Academy of Pediatrics (AAP) and the ACMG is that predictive genetic testing for late-onset disorders should not be performed unless there is a specific intervention during childhood that will reduce morbidity or mortality [53,54]. Also, the AAP does not support the broad use of carrier testing or screening in children or adolescents. As for any genetic testing, a medical benefit should be the primary justification for testing in children and adolescents. It is very important for parents to understand the limitations of testing before they sign informed consent for their children. The results of thrombophilia testing rarely influence medical management decisions and at the moment there is no evidence that thrombophilia testing could benefit a young healthy child. The incidence of venous thrombosis in healthy children is extremely low (0.07/100000), and the long-term use of anticoagulants in an asymptomatic healthy child would be unjustified [55].

Tormene et al. performed a prospective cohort study of children aged 1-14 years from families with a single identified inherited thrombophilia. The children were tested for FVL, prothrombin G20210A mutations and antithrombin, protein C and protein S deficiency and followed for the evidence of thrombosis 1-8 years (mean 5 years). No children with or without thrombophilia developed VTE during the study period [56]. Thrombophilia testing could show more benefit for children with the acute or chronic medical conditions. The overwhelming majority of pediatric TEs are associated with central venous lines (CVLs) [52].

Other acquired risk factors depend on the age of the child. Within the entire childhood population neonates are at the greatest risk of thromboembolism (5.1/100 000 live births per year in white children) [57]. Neonatal risk factors include birth asphyxia, respiratory distress syndrome, maternal diabetes, infections, necrotizing enterocolitis, dehydration, congenital nephrotic syndrome and polycythemia [57]. Children of any age may have antiphospholipid or anticardiolipin antibodies which are associated with thrombophilia [52]. Meta-analysis of Young et al. on impact of inherited thrombophilia on venous thromboembolism in children showed significant association with recurrent VTE for all inherited thrombophilia traits except the factor V variant and elevated lipoprotein (a) [58]. A second peak of incidence of thrombosis is during adolescence [59]. Adolescents may have the same risk factors as the adults including smoking, pregnancy, obesity, and oral contraceptives which increase the risk of thrombosis [52]. Adolescents identified with an inherited thrombophilia may benefit from avoiding high-risk situations (prolonged immobility, dehydration), pursuing healthy lifestyles (regular exercise and weight control), and recognizing early signs and symptoms of VTE [60].

There are some situations in which the presence of an inherited defect may influence medical decision making. The first is in an adolescent female who is interested in using oral contraceptive pills (OCPs). Knowledge of a congenital thrombophilia provide the opportunity to consider lower-risk alternatives for contraception, such as progesterone-only preparations. In limited cases, the presence of inherited thrombophilia might lead to targeted thrombophylaxis in high risk situations, e.g., after a femur fracture in an obese teenager, though there are few data to document the efficacy of this approach [60].

7. Genetic counseling

It is of major importance to provide genetic counseling to patients as well as to their asymptomatic family members who are interested in thrombophilia testing, including pharmacogenetic tests. Based on detailed information about a family history, personal history and the reasons for testing genetic counselor should provide education and support for the family members. During the pre-test genetic counseling patient or family member should understand that the testing is optional and that it will be performed only after signed informed consent. It must be clarified that this is a testing for susceptibility gene and not for the disease state and that an individual's thrombotic risk is determined by a complex interplay of genetic, acquired and circumstantial risk factors [1]. It must be clear to the family member that if thrombophilia mutation is inherited the risk of VTE is higher than it is in the general population but although the inheritance pattern is dominant the penetrance of the mutation is not 100%. In order to achieve a better understanding of potential risk when counseling a family member regarding the risk of thrombosis it is most useful to provide the absolute risk (e.g., incidence) of thrombosis among persons with particular thrombophilia [61]. Pre-test genetic counseling should include discussion not only about the risks but also about the benefits and limitations of testing for the patient and for the entire family. Asymptomatic family member should understand that testing for thrombophilia may have lower benefit to risk ratio as compared to symptomatic relative [62]. Post-test counseling is equally as important for family members who tested positive and negative. In case when the result is negative family members should understand that currently available tests might not identify all inherited risk factors for thrombosis [52]. In the other case discussion should include signs and symptoms of thrombosis, risk factors to avoid and the risks and benefits of prophylactic therapy [63]. Clinical geneticist should also be aware of psychological response of the tested individual. Results of the study of Louzada et al. do not support the concern that asymptomatic relatives are at risk of psychological distress as a consequence of thrombophilia screening [64]. However it is general conclusion that characteristics of the genetic predisposition, including the likelihood of developing the disease, perceived severity and availability of treatments for the condition are likely contributors to the psychological response [64]. It means that adequate genetic counseling is of key importance for education of family members, in order to increase their awareness of risk factors and effective interventions to prevent VTE.

As a conclusion, genetic tests are part of modern management and treatment of thrombophilia, but several medical and ethical dilemmas are still open. Healthcare professionals should apply evidence-based guidelines regarding indications for genetic and pharmacogenetic testing, as well as principles of genetic counseling in thrombophilia. In the upcoming era of personalized genomic medicine, genetic tests day after day become more available, but their real power and relevance is fully expressed in the context of clinical data.

Acknowledgements

This work was supported by Ministry of Education and Science, Republic of Serbia (Grant No. 175091).

Author details

Ivana Novaković[1], Nela Maksimović[1] and Dragana Cvetković[2]

1 Faculty of Medicine, University of Belgrade, Belgrade, Serbia

2 Faculty of Biology, University of Belgrade, Belgrade, Serbia

References

[1] Varga EA, Kujovich JL. Management of inherited thrombophilia: guide for genetics professionals. Clin Genet. 2012;81(1):7-17.

[2] Novaković I, Maksimovic N, Cvetkovic S, Cvetkovic D: Gene polymorphisms as markers of disease susceptibility. J Med Biochem., 2010;29(3):1-5.

[3] Novaković I, Cvetković D, Maksimović N: Inherited Thrombophilia and the risk of vascular events. in: Luigi Tranquilli A. (ed.): Thrombophilia. ISBN 978-953-307-872-4, InTech, Croatia, 2011, 59-74.

[4] Hellmann EA, Leslie ND, Moll S. Knowledge and educational needs of individuals with the factor V Leiden mutation. J Thromb Haemost. 2003;1(11):2335-9.

[5] Walker P, Gregg AR. Screening, testing, or personalized medicine: where do inherited thrombophilias fit best? Obstet Gynecol Clin North Am. 2010;37(1):87-107.

[6] Favaloro EJ, McDonald D, Lippi G. Laboratory investigation of thrombophilia: the good, the bad, and the ugly. Semin Thromb Hemost. 2009 Oct;35(7):695-710.

[7] American College of Medical Genetics. Principles of screening: report of the subcommittee of the American College ofMedical Genetics Clinical Practice Committee. http://www.acmg.net/resources/policies/pol-026.asp1997.

[8] Middeldorp S. Is thrombophilia testing useful? Hematology. American Society of Hematology Education Program Book. 2011;2011(1):150-5.

[9] Linkins LA, Choi PT, Douketis JD. Clinical impact of bleeding in patients taking oral anticoagulant therapy for venous thromboembolism: a meta-analysis. Ann Intern Med. 2003;139(11):893-900.

[10] Middeldorp S, Meinardi JR, Koopman MM, van Pampus EC, Hamulyak K, van Der Meer J, et al. A prospective study of asymptomatic carriers of the factor V Leiden mutation to determine the incidence of venous thromboembolism. Ann Intern Med. 2001;135(5):322-7.

[11] Coppens M, van de Poel MH, Bank I, Hamulyak K, van der Meer J, Veeger NJ et al. A prospective cohort study on the absolute incidence of venous thromboembolism and arterial cardiovascular disease in asymptomatic carriers of the prothrombin 20210A mutation. Blood 2006; 108(8):2604-7.

[12] Evaluation of Genomic Applications in Practice and Prevention (EGAPP) working group. Recommendations from the EGAPP Working Group: Routine testing for Factor V Leiden (R506Q) and prothrombin (20210G>A) mutations in adults with a history of idiopathic venous thromboembolism and their adult family members. Genetics in Medicine. 2011;13(1):67-76.

[13] Cushman M. Inherited Risk Factors for Venous Thrombosis. Hematology. American Society of Hematology Education Program Book. 2005;2005(1):452-7.

[14] Jekic B, Lukovic L, Bunjevacki V, Milic V, Novakovic I, Damnjanovic T, Milasin J, Popovic B, Maksimovic N, Damjanov N, Radunovic G, Kovacevic L, Krajinovic M. Association of the TYMS 3G/3G genotype with poor response and GGH 354GG genotype with the bone marrow toxicity of the methotrexate in RA patients. Eur J Clin Pharmacol. 2012 Jul 5. [Epub ahead of print], DOI 10.1007/s00228-012-1341-3

[15] Milic V, Jekic B, Lukovic L, Bunjevacki V, Milasin J, Novakovic I, Damnjanovic T, Popovic B, Maksimovic N, Damjanov N, Radunovic G, Pejnovic N, Krajinovic M. Association of dihydrofolate reductase (DHFR) -317AA genotype with poor response to methotrexate in patients with rheumatoid arthritis. Clin Exp Rheumatol. 2012;30(2): 178-83.

[16] Todorovic Z, Džoljić E, Novaković I, Mirković D, Stojanović R, Nešić Z, Krajinović M, Prostran M, Kostić V. Homocysteine serum levels and MTHFR C677T genotype in patients with Parkinson's disease, with and without levodopa therapy. J Neurol Sci. 2006; 248(1-2),56-61.

[17] Krcunović Z, Novakovic I, Maksimovic N, Bukvic D, Simic-Ogrizovic S, Jankovic S, Djukanovic L, Cvetkovic D. Genetic clues to the etiology of Balkan endemic nephropathy: Investigating the role of ACE and AT1R polymorphisms. Arch Biol Sci 2010;62(4),957-65.

[18] Pereira NL and Weinshilboum RM. Cardiovascular pharmacogenomics and individualized drug therapy. Nat Rev Cardiol. 2009; 6(10): 632–8.

[19] Damani SB, Topol EJ. Emerging clinical applications in cardiovascular pharmacogenomics. Wiley Interdiscip Rev Syst Biol Med. 2011; 3(2):206-15.

[20] Voora D, Ginsburg GS. Clinical application of cardiovascular pharmacogenetics. J Am Coll Cardiol. 2012; 60(1):9-20.

[21] Seip RL, Duconge J, Ruaño G. Implementing genotype-guided antithrombotic therapy. Future Cardiol. 2010; 6(3):409-24.

[22] Dumas TE, Hawke RL, Lee CR. Warfarin dosing and the promise of pharmacogenomics. Curr Clin Pharmacol. 2007; 2(1): 11-21.

[23] Takeuchi F, McGinnis R, Bourgeois S, Barnes C, Eriksson N, et al. A genome-wide association study confirms VKORC1, CYP2C9, and CYP4F2 as principal genetic determinants of warfarin dose. PLoS Genet. 2009; 5(3):e1000433.

[24] Higashi MK, Veenstra DL, Kondo LM, Wittkowsky AK, Srinouanprachanh SL et al. Association between CYP2C9 genetic variants and anticoagulation-related outcomes during warfarin therapy. JAMA 2002; 287(13):1690-8.

[25] Moyer TP, O'Kane DJ, Baudhuin LM, Wiley CL, Fortini A et al. Warfarin sensitivity genotyping: a review of the literature and summary of patient experience. Mayo Clin Proc. 2009; 84(12):1079-94.

[26] Singh O, Sandanaraj E, Subramanian K, Lee LH, Chowbay B. Influence of CYP4F2 rs2108622 (V433M) on warfarin dose requirement in Asian patients. Drug Metab Pharmacokinet. 2011; 26(2): 130-6.

[27] Daly AK. Optimal dosing of warfarin and other coumarin anticoagulants: the role of genetic polymorphisms. Arch Toxicol. 2013; 87:407–20.

[28] Suarez-Kurtz G, Botton MR. Pharmacogenomics of warfarin in populations of African descent. Br J Clin Pharmacol. 2013; 75(2): 334–46.

[29] Rieder MJ, Reiner AP, Gage BF, Nickerson DA, Eby CS et al. Effect of VKORC1 haplotypes on transcriptional regulation and warfarin dose. N Engl J Med. 2005; 352(22): 2285-93.

[30] Ross KA, Bigham AW, Edwards M, Gozdzik A et al. Worldwide allele frequency distribution of four polymorphisms associated with warfarin dose requirements. J Hum Genet. 2010; 55(9):582-9.

[31] Eckman MH, Rosand J, Greenberg SM, Gage BF. Cost-effectiveness of using pharmacogenetic information in warfarin dosing for patients with nonvalvular atrial fibrillation. Ann Intern Med. 2009; 150(2):73-83.

[32] Kovač M, Maslać A, Rakićević Lj, Radojković D. The c.-1639G>A polymorphism of the VKORC1 gene in Serbian population: retrospective study of the variability in response to oral anticoagulant therapy. Blood Coagulation & Fibrinolysis 2010; 21(6): 558–63.

[33] Kovač M, Rakićević Lj, Kusić-Tišma J, Radojković D. Pharmacogenetic tests could be helpful in predicting of VKA maintenance dose in elderly patients at treatment initiation. Journal of Thrombosis and Thrombolysis, 2012; DOI: 10.1007/s11239-012-0769-8.

[34] Zhang X, Li L, Ding X, Kaminsky LS. Identification of cytochrome P450 oxidoreductase gene variants that are significantly associated with the interindividual variations in warfarin maintenance dose. Drug Metab Dispos. 2011; 39(8): 1433-9.

[35] International Warfarin Pharmacogenetics Consortium, Klein TE, Altman RB, Eriksson N et al. Estimation of the warfarin dose with clinical and pharmacogenetic data. N Engl J Med 2009; 360(8):753-64.

[36] Sorich M, McKinnon R. Personalized Medicine: Potential, Barriers and Contemporary Issues. Current Drug Metabolism 2012; 13(7): 1000-6.

[37] Epstein RS, Moyer TP, Aubert RE, O'Kane DJ, Xia F et al. Warfarin Genotyping Reduces Hospitalization Rates. Results From the MM-WES (Medco-Mayo Warfarin Effectiveness Study). Journal of the American College of Cardiology 2010; 55 (25): 2804-12.

[38] Tormene D, Grandone E, De Stefano V, Tosetto A, Palareti G, Margaglione M, Castaman G, Rossi E, Ciminello A, Valdrè L, Legnani C, Tiscia GL, Bafunno V,Carraro S, Rodeghiero F, Simioni P. Obstetric complications and pregnancy-related venous thromboembolism: the effect of low-molecular-weight heparin on their prevention in carriers of factor V Leiden or prothrombin G20210A mutation. Thromb Haemost. 2012;107(3):477-84.

[39] Mitić G, Novakov Mikić A, Povazan L, Mitreski A, Kopitović V, Vejnović T. Thromboprophylaxis implementation during pregnancy in women with recurrent foetal losses and thrombophilia. Med Pregl. 2011;64(9-10):471-5.

[40] Marinov B, Pramatarova T, Andreeva A, Iarukova N, Slavov A. Our experience with management of inherited thrombophilia during pregnancy. Preliminary report. Akush Ginekol (Sofiia). 2011;50(6):15-7.

[41] de Jong PG, Goddijn M, Middeldorp S. Testing for inherited thrombophilia in recurrent miscarriage. Semin Reprod Med. 2011;29(6):540-7.

[42] Lund M, Nielsen HS, Hviid TV, Steffensen R, Nyboe Andersen A, Christiansen OB. Hereditary thrombophilia and recurrent pregnancy loss: a retrospective cohort study of pregnancy outcome and obstetric complications. Hum Reprod. 2010;25(12): 2978-84.

[43] Tang AW, Quenby S. Recent thoughts on management and prevention of recurrent early pregnancy loss. Curr Opin Obstet Gynecol. 2010;22(6):446-51.

[44] McNamee K, Dawood F, Farquharson RG. Thrombophilia and early pregnancy loss. Best Pract Res Clin Obstet Gynaecol. 2012;26(1):91-102.

[45] Coulam CB, Jeyendran RS, Fishel LA, Roussev R. Multiple thrombophilic gene mutations rather than specific gene mutations are risk factors for recurrent miscarriage. Am J Reprod Immunol. 2006;55(5):360-8.

[46] Simon A, Laufer N. Repeated implantation failure: clinical approach. Fertil Steril. 2012;97(5):1039-43.

[47] Ricci G, Bogatti P, Fischer-Tamaro L, Giolo E, Luppi S, Montico M, Ronfani L, Morgutti M. Factor V Leiden and prothrombin gene G20210A mutation and in vitro fertilization: prospective cohort study. Hum Reprod. 2011;26(11):3068-77.

[48] Rudick B, Su HI, Sammel MD, Kovalevsky G, Shaunik A, Barnhart K.Is factor V Leiden mutation a cause of in vitro fertilization failure? Fertil Steril. 2009;92(4):1256-9.

[49] Qublan H, Amarin Z, Dabbas M, Farraj AE, Beni-Merei Z, Al-Akash H, Bdoor AN,Nawasreh M, Malkawi S, Diab F, Al-Ahmad N, Balawneh M, Abu-Salim A. Low-molecular-weight heparin in the treatment of recurrent IVF-ET failure and thrombophilia: a prospective randomized placebo-controlled trial. Hum Fertil (Camb). 2008;11(4):246-53.

[50] Coulam CB, Jeyendran RS, Fishel LA, Roussev R. Multiple thrombophilic gene mutations are risk factors for implantation failure. Reprod Biomed Online. 2006;12(3): 322-7.

[51] Toth B, Würfel W, Germeyer A, Hirv K, Makrigiannakis A, Strowitzki T. Disorders of implantation--are there diagnostic and therapeutic options? J Reprod Immunol. 2011;90(1):117-23.

[52] Thornburg CD, Dixon N, Paulyson-Nunez K, Ortel T. Thrombophilia screening in asymptomatic children. Thrombosis Research.2008; 121:597-604.

[53] Nelson RM, Botkjin JR, Kodish ED, Levetown M, Truman JT, Wilfond BS, et al. Ethical issues with genetic testing in pediatrics. Pediatrics. 2001;107(6):1451–5.

[54] Points to consider: ethical, legal, and psychosocial implications of genetic testing in children and adolescents. American Society of Human Genetics Board of Directors, American College of Medical Genetics Board of Directors. Am J Hum Genet. 1995;57(5):1233–41.

[55] Andrew M, David M, Adams M, et al. Venous thromboembolic complications (VTE) in children: first analyses of the Canadian Registry of VTE. Blood. 1994;83:1251-7.

[56] Tormene D, Simioni P, Prandoni P, Franz F, Zerbinati P, Tognin G, et al. The incidence of venous thromboembolism in thrombophilic children: a prospective cohort study. Blood. 2002;100(7):2403–5.

[57] Nowak-Gottl U, Duering C, Kempf-Bielack B, Strater R. Thromboembolic diseases in neonates and children. Pathophysiol Haemost Thromb. 2003;33(5–6):269–74.

[58] Young G, Albisetti M, Bonduel M et al. Impact of Inherited Thrombophilia on Venous Thromboembolism in Children : A Systematic Review and Meta-Analysis of Observational Studies. Circulation. 2008;118:1373-82.

[59] Andrew M, Marzinotto V, Pencharz P, et al. A cross-sectional study of catheter-related thrombosis in children receiving total parenteral nutrition at home. J Pediatr. 1995;126:358-63.

[60] Raffini L. Thrombophilia in Children: Who to Test, How, When, and Why? Hematology. American Society of Hematology Education Program Book. 2008; 2008(1):228-35.

[61] Heit JA. Thrombophilia: Common Questions on Laboratory Assessment and Management. Hematology. American Society of Hematology. 2007; 127-35

[62] Reich LM, Bower M, Key NS. Role of the geneticist in testing and counseling for inherited thrombophilia. Genet Med 2003;5(3):133–43.

[63] College of American Pathologists Consensus Conference XXXVI: diagnostic issues in thrombophilia. Arch Pathol Lab Med 2002;126(11):1277–433.

[64] Louzada ML, Taljaard M, Langlois NJ. Psychological impact of thrombophilia testing in asymptomatic family members. Thrombosis Research. 2011;128:530-5.

Chapter 5

Thrombophilia in Systemic Lupus Erythematosus: A Review of Multiple Mechanisms and Resultant Clinical Outcomes

Patricia J. Dhar and Robert J. Sokol

Additional information is available at the end of the chapter

1. Introduction

Systemic lupus erythematosus, or SLE is a multisystem autoimmune disease that occurs predominantly in African American women of childbearing age, who generally have more severe disease. There are several multi-ethnic global lupus registries ongoing to collect better information on the epidemiology of SLE worldwide [1]. The annual incidence of SLE is 3 cases / 100,000 with prevalence rates reported up to 144/100,000 among the general population [1-2], 90% of SLE patients being female gender. African Americans and Hispanics as well as males with lupus, general ly have more severe diseases, particularly renal disease, with some studies also showing this association in Asians [1-2]. SLE is a thrombophilic state. Patients with SLE-related hypercoagulability can develop arterial and venous thrombosis as well as intrauterine fetal demise, such as miscarriages and stillbirths. Multiple mechanisms contribute to hyper-coagulability in SLE, including lupus specific factors such as antiphospholipid antibodies. These antibodies also contribute to cardiovascular and cerebrovascular disease in lupus. The inflammation in SLE can increase certain procoagulant factors which can tip the balance towards thrombosis. In addition, platelet hyperfunction in SLE promotes thrombogenesis and is particularly important in premature cardiovascular disease management in women with lupus. Thrombogenesis in SLE is best explained by the multiple-hit theory in which several procoagulant or anticoagulant effects occur, which additively can attain the critical overall effect needed to generate a blood clot. Thus, when assessing lupus patients for thrombosis or intrauterine fetal demise, a larger laboratory work up is needed to define the coagulation abnormalities in order to fine tune the most effective anticoagulation regimen as well as determine length of treatment. This chapter will briefly review the clinical syndromes associated with thrombophilic lupus related antibodies, with an emphasis on pregnancy loss, cardiovascular disease and clotting, the multiple mechanisms for hypercoagulability in SLE, and discuss the complexity of this problem in this population.

2. Epidemiology

2.1. Vascular thrombosis

The epidemiology of vascular thrombosis is well described in SLE and with several studies showing an increased risk for arterial and venous thrombosis. Arterial and venous thrombosis occurs in approximately 10% of SLE patients [3-7] with thrombosis being a major cause of death in patients with lupus [8]. Gender differences have been reported with male SLE patients having a higher prevalence of thrombosis and antiphospholipid antibody syndrome compared to women with lupus [9]. Thrombovascular events occur throughout the course of lupus disease with an increase risk over time [10-11]. Arterial vascular events occur more frequently in post-menopausal women with lupus and are associated with age, disease duration, smoking and mean dose of glucocorticoids [12]. Venous thrombosis is also associated with smoking in lupus [12]. Other risk factors for thrombosis in lupus include high disease activity, lupus nephritis /nephrotic syndrome, elevated homocysteine, and the presence of antiphospholipid antibodies [11, 13-16].

2.2. Pregnancy loss

The factors which increase thrombosis risk also promote pregnancy loss in lupus. Patients with SLE have increased frequencies of intrauterine growth restriction and fetal demise (miscarriage and stillbirth) which can predate the diagnosis of lupus [17-18]. Pregnancy complications in SLE are fairly common with maternal hypertensive complications occurring in 10-20%, preterm births in 20% and fetal growth restriction occurring in about 28%, with an average drop in fetal growth weight to be 16% [18-19]. Fetal wastage is markedly increased in SLE with stillbirths occurring in 4-22% and miscarriage rates reported to range from approximately 10-46% [18-19]. The increased stillbirth rate in SLE is 4 fold greater than the general population [18]. Intrauterine demise and adverse fetal outcome in SLE are related in great part to lupus specific thrombophilic factors, which can cause placental infarctions, decidual vasculopathy, and lower placental weight [20-22]. Placental histopathological findings in SLE patients with lupus anticoagulant or anti-cardiolipin antibodies include extensive infarctions due to decidual vasculopathy (related to fibrinoid necrosis in the wall of decidual arterioles and thrombosis), syncytial knots, and perivillous fibrinoid change [20-22]. In addition, there is a decrease in vasculo-syncytial membranes, an increase in fibrosis and an increase in hypovascular villi all which can lead to fetal growth restriction or demise [20-22]. Pregnancy itself is a hypercoagulable state with fetal demise, thrombosis and pre-eclampsia being related to Factor V Leiden mutation, prothrombin gene mutation 20210A, and deficiencies of anti-thrombin III, protein C and protein S [23]. Thus, SLE specific thrombophilic factors are additive to the background of pregnancy related hypercoagulability (multiple hits), and this increases the occurrence of adverse fetal outcomes in lupus.

2.3. Premature cardiovascular disease

Lupus-specific thrombophilic factors contribute to premature cardiac disease and atherosclerosis in this population. These lupus specific factors can affect the endothelium resulting in premature arterial vascular disease contributing to the accelerated/premature atherosclerosis observed in SLE [24]. Atheroma formation is initiated when oxidized low density lipoprotein (LDL) is taken up by foam cells in vascular endothelium [24-25]. High density lipoprotein (HDL) and Apo-A1 are protective factors against atherosclerosis. β-2 glycoprotein-1 binding to oxidized LDL facilitates uptake by foam cells [26]. Patients with SLE have antibodies to LDL/ β-2 glycoprotein-1 complexes, HDL, and Apo –A1 [26-27]. Antibodies to HDL and Apo A-1 cross react with cardiolipin and prevent HDL and Apo-1 protection against atherosclerosis. Antibodies to oxidized LDL may cross react with β-2 glycoprotein-1 and may enhance uptake, thus promoting plaque formation [25-28]. Anticardiolipin antibody binding exposes immunogenic and normally hidden (or cryptic) epitopes on β-2 glycoprotein-1, which can bind to anti- β-2 glycoprotein-1 antibodies. These antibodies bind to adhered β-2 glycoprotein-1 on endothelial cells which causes endothelial activation and subsequent up regulation of inflammatory and procoagulant factors [24-26]. In addition, adhered β-2 glycoprotein-1 on oxidized LDL promotes LDL uptake by macrophages, thus facilitating plaque formation [24-26, 28]. During the acute phase response, HDL can be converted to pro-inflammatory molecules which promote LDL oxidation. Chronic inflammation can cause HDL dysfunction in SLE. HDL has been found to be pro-inflammatory in women with SLE and is termed pro-inflammatory HDL or piHDL [25-26, 28]. More than 85% patients with SLE and carotid plaques had piHDL vs. 40% in those without plaques [27]. Pro- inflammatory HDL is an independent risk factor for atherosclerosis in rheumatoid arthritis and antiphospholipid antibody syndrome [26, 28]. The prevalence of moderate to severe atherosclerosis in SLE at autopsy is 52% [29]. There is a higher prevalence of coronary artery disease in SLE than general population which is not predicted by traditional risk factors or increase in lupus activity alone [30-39]. Mortality studies show coronary artery disease (CAD) /myocardial infarction (MI) is a frequent cause of death in SLE and occurs in 11-48% of SLE patients [3, 30-35]. Death from CAD in SLE is disproportionately larger in late disease, with CAD/MI being the leading cause of death in SLE survivors. This accounts for the late peak in mortality in SLE [36-38]. Although there are a greater number of CAD risk factors (hypertension, diabetes mellitus, dyslipidemia, sedentary life style) in SLE patients than matched controls, the increased atherosclerosis in SLE is not fully attributed to these traditional risk factors [39-41]. Several other studies have reported an increased risk of cardiovascular disease in SLE. After controlling for age, sex, cholesterol, hypertension, diabetes mellitus, tobacco use the relative risk was 10.1 for non-fatal myocardial infarction [95%, CI 5.8-15.6] and 17.0 for death due to coronary artery disease (CI 8.1-29.7) [42]. Esdaile also reported a 7.5X increased risk for developing coronary artery disease in SLE [42]. Progression of coronary artery calcification has been associated with age, cholesterol and smoking [43]. In particular, premenopausal aged women with lupus seem to have premature CAD with >50X increase in MI in SLE women 35-44 years, and the risk of cardiovascular events being 8-9 X increased in middle age SLE women [44-45]. We have also reported an increased risk of myocardial infarction in premenopausal women with SLE [46]. Thus, myocardial infarctions occur in patients with SLE at younger age than the general population, and using traditional risk factors alone is inadequate for developing prevention and treatment programs in asymptomatic SLE patients [42, 44].

2.4. Cerebrovascular disease

Cerebrovascular disease is increased in SLE with an increased risk of stroke reported to be 1.67, 3.2 and 7.9 X the general population [44, 47-48]. Age and hypertension are associated with progression of carotid intima media thickness and carotid artery plaque in SLE [43]. Male lupus patients tend to have a higher prevalence of strokes than females [49]. Antiphospholipid antibodies are established risk factors for ischemic stroke in lupus [50] and can increase cerebrovascular atherosclerotic disease [51].

3. Pathogenesis and mechanisms of hypercoagulability

3.1. Chronic inflammation

Chronic Inflammation, which occurs in SLE, contributes to the development of thrombosis and accelerated atherosclerosis [52]. Inflammation and infections are known epidemiologic risk factors for venous thrombosis [53]. Inflammation can cause an acquired thrombophilia and subsequent thrombosis [54]. Inflammation activates the procoagulant arm of the coagulation system and inhibits anticoagulation and fibrinolysis [55].There is an association of lupus disease activity (i.e., inflammation) and elevated erythrocyte sedimentation rate and/or C-reactive protein levels with vascular thrombosis. [5, 6, 56-57]. In fact, complement activation which occurs in lupus can promote thrombosis by activating the coagulation cascade at multiple levels [58]. It is well established that venous thrombosis can occur with elevated levels of procoagulant factors 2, 8, 9 and 10, as well as with decreased levels of anticoagulant factors (antithrombin 3, protein S and protein S [54]. Coagulation factors that increase with inflammation include Von Willebrand factor, fibrinogen, Factor VII, and Factor VIII. Increases in high sensitivity C –reactive protein (HSCRP), fibrinogen and factor VIII are in seen in lupus anticoagulant-related thrombosis [59]. Additionally, fibrinogen increases with time in SLE patients which may partially explain the increased risk of thrombosis with increasing years of lupus disease [11, 60]. Lupus disease activity is associated with elevated procoagulant markers thrombin-anti thrombin complexes, prothrombin fragment 1+2, and soluble thrombomodulin, suggesting inflammatory mediated hypercoagulability [61]. Inflammatory cytokines promote endothelial damage, plaque formation and vascular smooth muscle hypertrophy [62]. Pro-inflammatory cytokines which activate endothelial and vascular smooth muscle cells include interleukin 1 (IL-1), interleukin 6 (IL-6), tumor necrosis factor (TNF) and vascular endothelial growth factor (VEGF), all of which are increased in active lupus, particularly lupus nephritis [62]. CD 40 ligand is increased in lymphocytes in SLE patients and CD40/CD40 ligand interactions can cause plaque rupture [62]. Other pro-inflammatory effects which promote atherosclerosis include chemokines and adhesion molecules. Inflammation induces thrombosis via endothelial cell dysfunction, tissue factor mediated activation of coagulation, platelet activation, impaired function of anticoagulants and suppressed fibrinolytic activity [55]. These effects all play a role in venous thrombosis in lupus.

3.2. Hypercoagulability

Multiple mechanisms contribute to hypercoagulability in SLE and thrombosis is due to multiple hits to the clotting system (the multiple-hit theory). It has been shown that elevations of procoagulant factors in combination have an additive effect on thrombosis [63]. In lupus, this includes lupus-specific and non- specific thrombogenic factors. As discussed in the previous paragraph, inflammation can cause elevations of non- lupus related procoagulant factors. Other factors contributing to hypercoagulability in SLE includes hyperhomocysteine-mia [16, 64-66], and elevated plasminogen activator inhibitor-1 (PAI-1) which decreases fibrinolytic activity [16, 55], as well as deficiencies of anticoagulant factors such as protein C, protein S and tissue plasminogen activator (tPA)which activates the fibrinolytic system [17, 55]. Lupus-specific procoagulant factors include antiphospholipid antibodies. Other lupus-specific factors include antibodies to factor XII [67], prothrombin [68], and annexin V [69-71]. Antiphospholipid antibodies encompass anticardiolipin antibodies, lupus anticoagulant (LAC), anti- β-2 glycoprotein-1 antibodies and false positive rapid plasma reagin (RPR) tests. These antibodies are prevalent in SLE and are pathogenically involved in the thromboses, accelerated atherosclerosis and fetal demise seen in this population. The prevalence of antiphospholipid antibodies are common in SLE with anticardiolipin antibodies occurring in 17-86% (vs.1-6% in the general population), and LAC noted in 15-30% (vs. 1-4% in the general population) [72]. Antiphospholipid antibodies cause vascular thrombosis and fetal loss in SLE [6, 72-76]. The LAC has a much stronger association with venous thrombosis than anticardio-lipin antibodies where the thrombosis risk is directly related to increasing titers of these antibodies, particularly IGG anticardiolipin antibody titers of medium to high titer [5, 72, 77-78]. Low titers or transient presence of these antibodies generally do not cause thrombosis [72, 77]. These antibodies bind to phospholipids and protein epitopes found in cardiolipin, annexin V, prothrombin and β-2 glycoprotein-1 [24]. The antiphospholipid antibodies that recognize epitopes on β-2 glycoprotein-1 also bind serine proteases involved in hemostasis and fibrinolysis and hence promote thrombosis [79].

The prothrombotic effect of these antibodies occur via multiple mechanisms including platelet activation, endothelial cell activation with resultant up regulation of adhesion molecules and production of thromboxane A2, and stimulation of monocytes to make tissue factor, all of which promote clotting and vasoconstriction [80-81]. Tissue factor activates the extrinsic coagulation system while tissue plasminogen activator (tPA) activates fibrinolysis. Tissue factor pathway inhibitor activity is reduced in SLE and this is associated with increased levels of tissue factor and subsequent hypercoagulability [82]. Antiphospholipid antibodies bind to components of the coagulation cascade and activate the coagulation system leading to a procoagulant state along with decreased fibrinolysis via reducing activity of tPA [79-81].

Thrombosis and fetal loss in SLE share the same pathogenic pathways, and the mechanisms by which antiphospholipid antibodies cause fetal loss and thrombosis are complex and varied. They include target antigens in the coagulation, endothelial and immune systems summarized by Tripodi, et al, as follows [83]: 1.) inhibiting the protein C axis (targets- protein C, protein S, thrombomodulin, activated protein C ((APC) resistance, endothelial protein C receptor, 2.) increasing thrombin generation (targets- prothrombin, microparticles, tissue factor pathway inhibitor, protein Z, Factor XI, Factor XII, heparin cofactor II), 3.), disruption of the protective shield (target-annexin A5), 4.), decreasing fibrinolysis (targets-tPA, Annexin A2, β-2 glyco-protein-1 cleavage), 5.), altering complement levels (targets-C3, C5a, membrane attack complex, 6.) increasing platelet adhesion (target- Von Willebrand factor) and activation (targets-low density lipoprotein receptor 8, glycoprotein 1b, platelet factor 4, thromboxane A2, 7.) activation of endothelial cells (targets-Toll like receptor 4, tissue factor, prostacyclin, nitric oxide), 8.) activation of monocytes (target-tissue factor), 9.) activation of neutrophils (target-tissue factor), 10.) trophoblast activation (target-growth factor binding), 11.) angiogenesis (target- vascular endothelial growth factor, basic fibroblast growth factor), and 12.) increased atherosclerosis (target-oxidized LDL) [83-84]. In fact, β-2 glycoprotein-1 binds to oxidized LDL to form atherogenic complexes as discussed above. These complexes have been detected in patients with autoimmune disease and promote macrophage uptake and subsequent athero-sclerosis [85].

4. Laboratory diagnosis

Laboratory diagnosis of hypercoagulability in lupus is complex and depends on where the patient is in the disease process. In general, more than basic tests are needed to cover the full range of possibly disrupted clotting mechanisms and this includes testing for lupus specific antiphospholipid antibodies and other hemostatic markers of coagulation. The lupus-specific antibodies include lupus anticoagulant, anticardiolipin antibodies, and anti β-2 glycoprotein-1 antibodies. These antiphospholipid antibodies are a heterogeneous group of antibodies identified by various laboratory tests all of which have some problems with standardization, specificity, interpretation and quality control [86-89]. The target antigens for these antibodies include prothrombin, negatively charged phospholipids (such as phosphatidic acid, phos-phatidylinositol and phophatidyl serine), protein C, protein S, Annexin V, β-2 glycoprotein-1, thrombomodulin, factor XII, platelet adhesive receptor glycoprotein GP 1b (which binds Von Willebrand factor) and other factors mentioned above [81, 86-90]. Anticardiolipin antibodies are directed against a protein known as β-2 glycoprotein-1, which binds anionic phospholipids [86-87]. Lupus anticoagulants encompass a heterogeneous group of antibodies that bind negatively charged phospholipids. The assay for LAC is a functional assay which measures the activity of these antibodies [84]. Anticardiolipin antibodies bind directly to cardiolipin as well as β-2 glycoprotein-1 bound to cardiolipin, and are generally detected by enzyme-linked immunosorbent assay or ELISA [69]. A subgroup of these anticardiolipin antibodies bind β-2 glycoprotein-1, and it is these anticardiolipin antibodies that are pathogenic for thrombosis. β-2 glycoprotein-1 is a glycoprotein found on many cells including endothelial cells, astrocytes, neurons, extravillous cytotrophoblasts, and syncytiotrophoblast cells of the placenta [84]. β-2 glycoprotein-1 has five domains of which domain V binds anionic phospholipids. Antibodies to domain I seem to be the most important domain related to thrombosis [84, 87]. The anti β-2 glycoprotein-1 antibodies are considered a "cofactor" for anticardiolipin antibody activity but are essentially a more specific assay for evaluation of clinically relevant prothrombotic antiphospholipid antibodies [87].

Detection of these antiphospholipid antibodies by current testing is problematic due to variable performance in different laboratories as well as difficulty of standardization [83, 86-87]. The recommended method for detecting lupus anticoagulant is a functional assay and involves a 3 step process: 1) *Screening* via dilute Russel viper venom time or dRVVT and activated partial thromboplastin time or APTT, and if results are above normal (i.e., prolonged dRVVT or APTT) proceed to 2.) *Mixing* 1:1 of patient: pooled normal plasma and repeat testing. If results show that the clotting time (dRVVT and APPT) is still prolonged (i.e., not corrected), then proceed to 3.) *Confirmatory* step, which is to repeat testing with excess phospholipids. LAC is present if the confirmatory step shows correction of the clotting time since the LAC will bind the excess phospholipids and not the coagulation factors [83]. Anticardiolipin antibodies and anti β-2 glycoprotein-1 antibodies are both measured by ELISA. For anticardiolipin antibodies, there are specific protocols and guidelines for performing this test with some disagreement about positivity for cut off values at the lower titers [86-87, 91]. The anti β-2 glycoprotein-1 antibody tests are also done by ELISA but are more specific than the anticardiolipin antibody ELISA test, due to having a well-defined antigen (β-2 glycoprotein-1) for this assay, and is more consistent between different laboratories. [86-87]. It is currently recommended that all three assays be done for evaluation antiphospholipid antibodies in SLE and patients classified by number and type of tests positive, with the highest risk for thrombosis being in those with positive for all three tests and particularly with the immunoglobulin G or IgG isotype [83]. Much work still needs to be done to improve standardization, validity and consistency of test positivity between laboratories.

Along with the antiphospholipid antibodies discussed above which must be measured in patients with thrombosis or fetal loss in lupus patients with thrombosis or fetal loss, other hemostatic markers should be measured to better assess coagulation risk in SLE, i.e., a coagulation risk laboratory profile. This includes a broad panel of testing to include fibrinogen, factor VII, factor VIII, tPA, PAI-1, plasminogen activity, Von Willebrand factor activity and antigen, protein S activity, protein C activity homocysteine, and high sensitivity C-reactive protein or HSCRP [16]. It is also important to remember that estrogens and pregnancy can induce protein S deficiency and this may compound pregnancy and hormonal therapy management in lupus. Homocysteine has been associated with thrombosis in SLE, and should be measured in lupus patients as part of any hypercoagulable work up [16, 92-94]. Interestingly, rheological evaluation of SLE patients with and without thrombosis showed no association of blood viscosity and erythrocyte aggregation with thrombosis [95].

Congenital coagulation factors have been studied in in a limited fashion in SLE. The MTHFR 677 C>T polymorphism is associated with elevated homocysteine. This polymorphism was found to be homozygous form in 16.7% and heterozygous form in 83.3% of SLE patients tested and the homozygous form was increased in SLE patients vs. controls [57]. On the other hand, Factor V Leiden and Prothrombin G20210AS gene polymorphisms were not increased in SLE patients with thrombosis [64, 94]. These 2 gene polymorphisms are generally seen in Northern

European Caucasian populations so it is not surprising that SLE populations, being more predominantly African American, would not show any increase of these gene types. The PROFILE cohort study by Kaiser, et al, assessed 33 single nucleotide polymorphisms (SNPs) in 1,361 predominantly Caucasian SLE patients and found that genetic risk factors for thrombosis in this cohort differed across ethnic groups, and there was an association of venous thrombosis and SNPs for these genes in whites for Factor V Leiden (OR=2.69, p=0.002), for MTHFR (OR=1.51, p=0.01), and for fibrinogen gamma (OR=1.49, p=0.02) [96]. Evaluation of functional polymorphisms of the coagulation Factor II gene, which is associated with elevated levels and activity of prothrombin and thrombosis, showed an association of one particular polymorphism (rs313516 G allele) with SLE susceptibility in African Americans and Caucasians [97]. Micro-RNAs are non-coding RNAs which function to control gene regulation post transcription by regulating mRNA translation or stability. One study assessing micro-RNAs in SLE showed that specific micro-RNAs resulted in increased tissue factor production and increased procoagulant activity [98]. There is limited data on PAI-1 promoter 4G/5G polymorphisms in SLE. Increased PAI-1 activity is associated with reduced endogenous fibrinolytic activity and is a risk factor for thrombosis. The 4G/4G genotype for PAI-1 promoter has the highest levels of PAI-1 activity and hence the highest risk for thrombosis. SLE patients with the4G/4G genotype were found to have increased carotid atherosclerosis [99]. In addition, SLE patients with PAI-1 4G/4G homozygosity were at increased risk for glomerular microthrombi [100]. An additional risk factor for the development of arterial thrombosis in antiphospholipid antibody syndrome is the presence of the 4G allele of the 4G/5G polymorphism of the PAI-1 gene [101].

5. Platelet function in SLE

Although platelet hyperfunction plays an important role in thrombosis in SLE, it has not been well studied in this population. There is some evidence that platelet activation occurs in SLE and is associated with thrombosis [102-105]. Platelet hyperfunction and platelet activation can be induced by inflammation or antiphospholipid antibodies [106-108]. Antiphospholipid antibodies have been shown to bind to β-2 glycoprotein-1 -phospholipid complexes on activated platelet membranes. Sticky platelet syndrome or hyperfunctioning platelets is a well described autosomal dominant disorder associated with arterial and venous thrombosis and characterized by hyperaggregable platelets in response to adenosine diphosphate (ADP), epinephrine or both [109-111]. Hyperaggregable platelets have been described in other conditions including diabetes, unstable angina, atrial fibrillation, thrombotic strokes, migraine headaches, retinal artery occlusions, pre-eclampsia, arterial thromboembolism, nephrotic syndrome and patients in intensive care units [109-111]. This suggests that platelet aggregation is a response to stress or epinephrine [109-111]. In women with recurrent miscarriages, sticky platelet syndrome was found in 21% [112]. Enhanced platelet aggregation was noted in non-lupus patients with venous thromboembolism [113]. It is logical to assume that SLE patients would have activated platelets and platelet hyperfunction due to stress, inflammation and antiphospholipid antibody mediated activation. Few studies have assessed platelet function in SLE. Platelet activation markers CD 62 and CD 63 are increased in patients with primary antiphospholipid antibody syndrome, suggesting platelet activation plays an important role in thrombosis mediated by antiphospholipid antibodies [114]. *In vitro* platelet activation measured by flow cytometry using anti CD 62 was augmented by the presence of lupus plasma samples containing anticardiolipin antibodies and LAC [115]. Persistent activation of platelets (measured by platelet induced extracellular phosphorylation of plasma proteins) was seen in lupus patients, particularly those with thrombosis but not in non-SLE patients with DVT [116]. Our study (Dhar, et al) showed that 70% of SLE patients who had a hypercoaguable state had hyperfunctioning platelets measured by a functional assay [16].

Platelet hypofunction can also occur in SLE and has also not been well studied. Platelet hypofunction is usually the result of platelet dense granule deficiency and can result in bleeding and bruising disorders. Prolonged bleeding times suggesting platelet hypofunction have been described lupus patients who had LAC [117]. Our study (Dhar, et al) showed that the patients who had bleeding problems had platelet dense granule deficiency as measured by electron microscopy [16].

6. Approach to patients: Work up and thrombophilia management

6.1. High risk clinical scenarios

Selecting SLE patients for a coagulation assessment is well established for those with a thrombosis or fetal loss but is not well defined for those who are at risk but have not yet had an event. Thus, patients who have had an event should clearly be selected for a coagulation work up. The guidelines for this are the Sydney Clinical Criteria for antiphospholipid antibody syndrome [118]. This includes any 1.) vascular (arterial, venous or small vessel) thrombosis except for superficial thrombosis, 2.) Pregnancy morbidity (one or more unexplained deaths of a morphologically normal fetus at or beyond 10 weeks of gestation, one or more premature births of a morphologically normal neonate at or before 34 weeks gestation due to severe pre-eclampsia, eclampsia or severe placental insufficiency, or three or more unexplained consec-utive spontaneous abortions before the 10th week of gestation excluding anatomic or hormonal abnormalities or maternal/paternal chromosomal causes [118]. However, medical manage-ment should advance towards prevention of thrombosis and adverse fetal outcomes and one should evaluate high risk clinical settings as reason enough for a thrombophilic risk assess-ment. These would include pregnancy, pre-estrogen hormone therapy, pre-tamoxifen therapy, pre-organ transplant, pre- vascular procedure (such as coronary artery stenting), pulmonary hypertension, nephrotic syndrome, and chronic inflammatory setting, etc. In other words, one should assess the risk of thrombosis in the clinical situation and assess the multiple hits on that background. If the clinical setting is high risk for thrombophilia, one should do the coagulation profile discussed above along with genetics and platelet function studies. Then once this information is obtained, one should assess the number and degree of procoagulant hits and determines a treatment plan. This allows fine tuning of treatment while minimizing bleeding risk. Treatment strategies should be tailored to minimize bleeding complications, reduce recurrence of thrombosis, reduce intrauterine fetal demise, and simplify monitoring. Another complicating issue for thrombophilia management is that SLE patients frequently have mixed disorders with both prothrombotic and bleeding tendencies. Thus, when ordering a laboratory work up, an extensive battery of tests is needed to most accurately define the coagulation status. Unfortunately, since these factor abnormalities are independent of each other for the most part, there is no way to truncate the testing to an algorithm. However, as much information as possible should be obtained to determine the procoagulant and anticoagulant factors that would increase the risk for thrombosis and decide on optimal treatment.

6.2. Thromboprophylaxis for hypercoagulable states

For those SLE patients with hypercoagulability who have not had a thrombosis, treatment options for hypercoagulability in lupus consist of thromboprophylaxis for acute high risk situations, chronic prophylaxis for thrombosis prevention, and full dose anticoagulation therapy. Thromboprophylaxis for patients without any history of thrombosis and presence of antiphospholipid antibodies is controversial. However, evaluating thrombosis risk by assessing the multiple hits with a full thrombophilia profile would provide more support for deciding on intensity and type of thromboprophylactic treatment. High risk settings for which acute/short term thromboprophylaxis is indicated for antiphospholipid antibody positive patients would include surgery, ovarian stimulation or other short term hormonal therapy, pregnancy, vascular procedures, lupus flares, infections, and prolonged immobilization [119]. In pregnant SLE patients positive for lupus anticoagulant, it is recommended that low dose molecular weight or unfractionated heparin be used during pregnancy since neiher cross the placenta [19]. It is not recommended to treat thrombophilia in pregnant SLE patients who are positive for anti cardiolipin antibodies or lupus anticoagulant with corticosteroids since only anticoagulation has been shown to be of proven benefit in preventing thrombosis and fetal loss [19]. Corticosteroids have no benefit in preventing thrombotic complications in this setting and should only be used if any active lupus disease is present [19]. In addition, there is no role for prophylactic corticosteroids in patients who have no active lupus disease. Corticosteroids are relatively safe to use during pregnancy from a fetal standpoint, since the placenta metabolizes 90 % of non-flourinated corticosteroids. However, corticosteroids increase maternal complications such as hypertension and gestational diabetes [19]. Appropriate settings for chronic thromboprophylaxis would include those patients with persistent medium to high titers of anticardiolipin antibodies, those with triple antiphospholipid antibody positivity (+LAC, +anticardiolipin antibody, and +anti β-2 glycoprotein-1 antibody), and those with multiple hits on a background of high risk clinical settings such as, long term hormonal therapy, nephrotic syndrome, cardiovascular disease, and history of obstetric antiphospholipid antibody related events [119]. Both platelet function and the balance of procoagulant and anticoagulant factors should be assessed. Low dose aspirin therapy for prophylaxis is recommended by the Task Force at the 13th International congress on Antiphospholipid Antibodies for these aforementioned situations along with lifestyle changes and is commonly accepted as standard treatment by many [120-121]. In SLE patients with antiphospholipid antibodies, the task force recommends both low dose aspirin and hydroxychloroquine [120]. In pregnant SLE patients with antiphospholipid antibodies only and no previous history of pregnancy loss, low dose aspirin is recommended [122]. If platelet hyperfunction is present, low dose aspirin is indicated. If hyperhomocysteinemia is present, folic acid and B complex should be used to lower homocysteine levels to below 10 μmoles/liter. However, if other high risk situations are identified in which thrombosis is likely, such as very low protein S activity, then anticoagulation with warfarin or low molecular weight heparin is indicated.

6.3. Treatment of hypercoagulable states with prior vascular thrombosis

For those SLE patients with antiphospholipid antibodies and hypercoagulablity who have had an arterial or venous thrombosis full dose anticoagulation is recommended with unfractionated or low molecular weight heparin (e.g., enoxaparin, dalteparin), fondaparinux (a synthetic of the minimal anti thrombin binding sequence of heparin), vitamin K antagonists (e.g., warfarin), direct thrombin inhibitors (e.g., dabigatran), or direct factor Xa inhibitors (e.g., rivaroxaban) [83, 123]. For acute arterial or venous thrombosis, treatment consists of an initial course of unfractionated or low molecular weight heparin followed by indefinite long term treatment with warfarin to keep the international normalized ration or INR between 2.0-3.0, heparin- type drugs, or more recently, one of the newer thrombin or factor Xa inhibitors. For arterial thrombosis (stroke, myocardial infarction), addition of antiplatelet agents (low dose aspirin, clopidogrel 75 mg) may be helpful, particularly if platelet hyperfunction is present [16, 83]. The disadvantage of using warfarin is the difficulty of maintaining the correct therapeutic INR range and frequency of INR testing that must be done, which is inconvenient to the patient. The disadvantage of the heparin- type drugs is that the patient must administer self-injections daily. The heparin- type drugs do have one advantage in that coagulation lab monitoring is unnecessary. The newer thrombin or factor Xa inhibitor drugs have the dual advantage of being an oral medication and not requiring laboratory anticoagulation monitoring. For catastrophic antiphospholipid antibody syndrome, which has a high mortality rate, treatment with plasma exchange, high dose corticosteroids, intavenous immunoglobulins and anticoagulation is recommended [124].

6.4. Pregnancy

SLE pregnancies should be considered high risk and must be managed in a multidisciplinary setting to address three problem areas: hypertensive pregnancy complications, lupus disease activity and thrombophilia [19]. Pregnancy is a hypercoagulable state which is worsened by the inflammation of active lupus disease. Pregnancy outcomes are worse with active lupus, particularly nephritis and active central nervous system (CNS) disease. Thus, it is recommended that patients with SLE have planned pregnancies and not attempt conception until the disease has been in remission for the preceeding 6 months [19]. Pregnancies that occur during active lupus or in patients with a history of severe major organ involvement such as nephritis or CNS disease are higher risk for poor fetal outcomes and maternal complication [19].Patients with mild disease generally have good pregnancy outcomes. For those pregnant SLE patients with no prior pregnancy loss or previous vascular thrombosis who have anti phospholipid antibodies, it is recommended that prophylaxis with low dose aspirin be used [125]. However if there are multiple hits such as triple antiphospholipid antibody positivity, low dose aspirin along with prophylactic doses of unfractionated or low molecular weight heparin be used [125-126]. Pregnancy- induced protein S deficiency can occur in these patients and when present should be treated with full dose anticoagulation with of unfractionated or low molecular weight heparin to prevent pregnancy loss. For pregnant SLE patients with antiphospholipid antibodies, other hypercoagulability factors, and a previous pregnancy loss or vascular thrombosis, treatment with full dose of unfractionated or low molecular weight heparin along with dose aspirin is recommended [127-128]. Generally anticoagulation is interrupted briefly during the delivery period and resumed and continued post- partum until the protein S levels return to normal and the other coagulation parameters correct. For antiphospholipid antibody persistence post-partum, continued treatment with daily aspirin is often used. Although these treatments for pregnant SLE patients are generally accepted, there is a lack of definitive data from clinical trials to support these accepted regimens [83].

6.5. Adjuvant treatments

Other adjuvant treatments summarized by Mehudi [81] for antiphosphoipid antibodies in SLE include: 1.) statins (which decrease antiphospholipid antibody mediated thrombosis and inflammation, 2.)Ritxuamib (which depletes CD 20 B lymphocyte cells involved in antiphospholipid antibodyl mediated disease), 3.) Hydroxychloroquine (which inhibit platelet aggregation of antiphospholipid- activated platelets by binding to GPIIbIIIa and by binding β-2 glycoprotein-1 or to target cells), 4.) Specific GPIIbIIIa inhibitors (e.g,abciximb) which bind and inactivate GPiia IIIb which is upregulated on antiphospholipid antibody activated platelets, 5.) inhibitors of tissue factor up regulation seen in antiphopholipid antibody activated endothelial cells (e.g., ACE inhibitors), 6.) anti TNF therapy to block high TNF levels seen in antiphospholipid antibody positive patients, 7.) blockage of receptors for β-2 glycoprotein-1 or antiphospholipid antibodies on target cells [81].

7. Conclusion

It is clear that thrombophilia assessment and management is complex in SLE. The balance of procoagulant factors, anticoagulant factors and platelet function determine the overall hypercoagulability risk. Simply testing for antiphospholipid antibodies alone is inadequate for determining thrombophilia status and risk in SLE. Extended coagulation profile testing along with genetic evaluation of procoagulant markers and measurements of platelet function provide more clear and precise information to develop a thrombotic or fetal loss risk assessment in SLE. This allows for fine tuning of prophylactic or full dose anticoagulation treatment and may help determine intensity and length of treatment. The overall benefit of this extended testing is to improve selection of patients to treat, improve management of anticoagulation therapy, reduce re-thrombosis and fetal loss risk, and minimize treatment complications. Further research is needed to better elucidate the multiple mechanisms behind hypercoagulability in lupus with thrombotic risk stratification and subsequent development of more definitive treatment recommendations.

Author details

Patricia J. Dhar and Robert J. Sokol

Wayne State University School of Medicine, Departments of Internal Medicine and Obstetrics & Gynecology, Division of Rheumatology, C.S. Mott Center for Human Growth and Development, Detroit, Michigan, USA

References

[1] Villa-Blanco I, Calvo-Alen J. Utiliizing Registries in Systemic Lupus Erythematosus Clinical Research. Expert Rev 2012; 8(4): 353-360

[2] Feldman, CH, Hiraki LT, Liu J, Fischer MA, Solomon DH, Alarcon GS, Winkelmayer WC, Costenbader KH. Arthritis and Rheumatism 2013; 65(3); 753-763.

[3] Cervera R, Khamashta MA, Font J, Sepastiani GD, Gil A, Lavilla P, Meja JC, Aydintug AO, Chwalinska-Sadowska H, de Ramon E, Fernandez-Nebro A, Galeazzi M, Valen M, Mathieu A, Houssiau F, Caro N, Alba P, Ramon-Casals M, Ingelmo M, Hughes GR; European Working Party on Systemic Lupus Erythematosus. Morbidity and mortality in systemic lupus erythematosus during a 10-year period: a comparison of early and late manifestations in a cohort of 1,000 patients. Medicine (Baltimore) 2003; 82: 299-308.

[4] Sarabi ZS, Chang E, Bobba R, Ibanez D, Gladman D, Urowitz M, Forin PR. Incidence rates of aterial and venous thrombosis after diagnosis of systemic lupus erythematosus. Arthritis and Rheumatism 2005; 53: 609-12.

[5] Calvo-Alen J, Toloza SMA, Fernandez M, Bastian HM, Fessler BJ, Roseman JM, McGwin G, Vila LM, Reveille JD, Alarcon GS for the LUMINA Study Group. Systemic lupus erythematosus in a multiethnic US cohort (LUMINA): XXV, Smoking, older age, disease activity, lupus anticoagulant, and glucocorticoid dose as risk factors for the occurrence of venous thrombosis in lupus patients. Arthritis and Rheumatism 2005; 52: 2060-8.

[6] Toloza SMA, Uribe AG, McGwin G, Alacron GS, Fessler BJ, Bastian HM, Vila LM, Wu R, Shoenfeld Y, Roseman JM, Reveille JD for the LUMINA Study Group. Systemic lupus erythematosus in a multiethnic US cohort (LUMINA); XXIII, Baseline predictors of vascular events. Arthritis and Rheumatism 2004; 50: 3947-57.

[7] Calvo-Alen J, Alarcon GS, Tew MB, Tan FK, McGwin G, Fessler BJ, Vila LM, Reveille JD for the LUMINA Study Group. Systemic lupus erythematosus in a multiethnic US cohort. XXXIV, Deficient mannose-binding lectin exon 1 polymophisms are associated with cerebrovascular but not with other arterial thrombotic events. Arthritis and Rheumatism 2006; 54: 1940-5.

[8]   Cervera R, Khamashta MA, Font J, Sebastiani GD, Gil A, Lavilla P, Aydintug AO, Je-dryka-Góral A, de Ramón E, Fernández-Nebro A, Galeazzi M, Haga HJ, Mathieu A, Houssiau F, Ruiz-Irastorza G, Ingelmo M, Hughes GR. Morbidity and mortality in systemic lupus erythematosus during a 5-year period. A multicenter prospective study of 1,000 patients. European Working Party on Systemic Lupus Erythematosus. Medicine (Baltimore). 1999 May;78(3):167-75

[9]   Stefanidou, S, Benos,A, Galanopoulou,V, Chatziyannis,I, Kanakoudi,F, Aslanidis, S, Boura,P, Sfetsios,T, Settas,T, Katsounaros,M, Papadopoulou, D, Giamalis, P,Dom-bros, Chatzistilianou, N, Garyfallos, AClinical expression and morbidity of systemic lupus erythematosus during a post-diagnostic 5-year follow-up: a male:female com-parison. Lupus (2011) 20, 1090–1094.

[10] Chang ER., Pineau CA, Bertansky S, Neville C, Clarke AE, Portin PR. Risk for inci-dent arterial or venous vascular events varies over the course of systemic lupus er-ythematosus. J Rheumatol. 2006; 33(9):1780-4

[11] Somers E, Mager LS, Petri M. Antiphospholipid antibodies and incidence of throm-bosis in a cohort of patients with systemic lupus erythematosus. J Rheumatol 2002; 29: 2531-6.

[12] Fernandez M, Calvo-Alen J, Alarcon GS, Roseman JM, Bastian HM, Fesler BJ, McGwin G, Vila LM, Sanchez ML. Reveille JD for the LUMINA study group. System-ic lupus erythematosus in a multiethnic US cohort (LUMINA). XXI. Disease activity, damage accrual, and vascular events in pre- and postmenopausal women. Arthritis and Rheumatism 2005;52: 1655-64.

[13] Burgos PI, Alarcón GS. Thrombosis in systemic lupus erythematosus:risk and protec-tion. Expert Rev Cardiovasc Ther 2009; 7:1541-9.

[14] Sallai KK, Nagy E, Bodo I, Mohl A, Gergely P. Thrombosis risk in systemic lupus er-ythematosus: the role of thrombophilic riskfactors. Scand J Rheumatol 2007; 36: 198-205.

[15] Martínez-Berriotxoa A, Ruiz-Irastorza G, Egurbide MV, Rueda M, Aguirre C. Homo-cysteine, antiphospholipid antibodies and risk of thrombosis in patients with system-ic lupus erythematosus. Lupus 2004; 13: 927-33.

[16] Dhar JP, Andersen J, Essenmacher L, Ager J, Sokol RJ. Thrombophilic Patterns of Co-agulation Factors in Systemic Lupus Erythematosus. Lupus 2009;18; 400.

[17] Yasmeen S, Wilkins EE, Field NT, Sheikh RA, Gilbert WM. Pregnancy outcomes in women with systemic lupus erythematosus. J Matern Fetal Med. 2001 Apr;10(2):91-6

[18] Dhar JP, Essenmacher L, Ager J, Sokol RJ. Pregnancy Outcomes Before and After Di-agnosis of Systemic Lupus Erythematosus: American Journal of Obstetrics & Gyne-cology: 193; 1444-55, 2005.

[19] Dhar, JP, Sokol RJ. Lupus and Pregnancy: Complex Yet Manageable. Clinical Medicine & Research 2006; 4(4): 310-320.

[20] Ogishima D, Matsumoto T, Nakamura Y, Yoshida K, Kuwabara Y. Placental pathology in systemic lupus erythematosus with antiphospholipid antibodies. Pathol Int. 2000 Mar;50(3):224-9.

[21] Out HJ, Kooijman CD, Bruinse HW, Derkson RHWM. Histopathological Findings in Placentae from Patients with Intra-uterine Fetal Death and Anti-phospholipid Antibodies. European Journal of Obstetrics & Gynecology and Reproductive Biology 1991; 41: 179-186.

[22] Arias F, Romero R, Joist H, Kraus FT. Thrombophilia: a Mechanism of Disease in Women with Adverse Pregnancy Outcome and Thrombotic Lesions in the Placenta. J Matern Fetal Med 1998; 7(6): 277-286.

[23] Arkel YS, Ku DH.Thrombophilia and pregnancy: review of the literature and some original data.Clin Appl Thromb Hemost. 2001 Oct;7(4):259-68.

[24] Feinbloom D, Bauer K. Assessment of hemostatic risk factors in predicting arterial thrombotic events. Arteriosclerosis, Thrombosis, and Vascular Biology 2005; 25: 2043-53.

[25] Goyal T, Mitra S, Khaidakov M, Wang X, Singla S, Ding Z, Liu S, Mehta JL. Current Concepts of the Role of Oxidized LDL Receptors in Atherosclerosis. Curr Atheroscler Rep. 2012 Jan 29. (Epub ahead of print)

[26] Hahn BH, McMahon M. Atherosclerosis and systemic lupus erythematosus: the role of altered lipids and of autoantibodies. Lupus. 2008 May;17(5):368-70.

[27] McMahon M, Grossman J, Skaggs B, Fitzgerald J, Sahakian L, Ragavendra N, Charles-Schoeman C, Watson K, Wong WK, Volkmann E, Chen W, Gorn A, Karpouzas G, Weisman M, Wallace DJ, Hahn BH. Dysfunctional proinflammatory high-density lipoproteins confer increased risk of atherosclerosis in women with systemic lupus erythematosus. Arthritis Rheum. 2009 Aug;60(8):2428-37.

[28] Hahn BH, Grossman J, Chen W, McMahon M.The pathogenesis of atherosclerosis in autoimmune rheumatic diseases: roles of inflammation and dyslipidemia.J Autoimmun. 2007 Mar-May;28(2-3):69-75. Epub 2007 Apr 16.

[29] Abu-Shakra M, Urowitz MB, Gladman DD, Gough J.Mortality studies in systemic lupus erythematosus. Results from a single center. I. Causes of death.J Rheumatol. 1995 Jul;22(7):1259-64.

[30] Urowitz MB, Gladman DD, Tom BD, Ibañez D, Farewell VT. Changing patterns in mortality and disease outcomes for patients with systemic lupus erythematosus. J Rheumatol. 2008 Nov;35(11):2152-8. Epub 2008 Sep 15.

[31] Gustafsson J, Simard JF, Gunnarsson I, Elvin K, Lundberg IE, Hansson LO, Larsson A, Svenungsson E. Risk factors for cardiovascular mortality in patients with systemic

lupus erythematosus, a prospective cohort study.Arthritis Res Ther. 2012 Mar 5;14(2):R46. (Epub ahead of print)

[32] Doria A, Iaccarino L, Ghirardello A, Zampieri S, Arienti S, Sarzi-Puttini P, Atzeni F, Piccoli A, Todesco S. Long-term prognosis and causes of death in systemic lupus erythematosus. Am J Med. 2006 Aug;119(8):700-6.

[33] Chambers SA, Allen E, Rahman A, Isenberg D. Damage and mortality in a group of British patients with systemic lupus erythematosus followed up for over 10 years. Rheumatology (Oxford). 2009 Jun;48(6):673-5. Epub 2009 Apr 9.

[34] Björnådal L, Yin L, Granath F, Klareskog L, Ekbom A.Cardiovascular disease a hazard despite improved prognosis in patients with systemic lupus erythematosus: results from a Swedish population based study 1964-95. J Rheumatol. 2004 Apr;31(4): 713-9.

[35] Souza DC, Santo AH, Sato EI. Mortality profile related to systemic lupus erythematosus: a multiple cause-of-death analysis.J Rheumatol. 2012 Mar;39(3):496-503. Epub 2012 Jan 15.

[36] Rubin, LA, Urowitz MB, Gladmann DD. Mortality in systemic lupus erythematosus:the bimodal pattern revisited. Q J Med 1985: 55: 87-98

[37] Urowitz MB, Bookman AAM, Koehler BE, Gordan DA, Smythe HA, Ogryzlo MA: the bimodal mortality pattern of systemic lupus erythematosus. Am J Med 1976; 60: 221-5

[38] Symmons DP, Gabriel SE.Epidemiology of CVD in rheumatic disease, with a focus on RA and SLE. Nat Rev Rheumatol. 2011 May 31;7(7):399-408. doi: 10.1038/nrrheum. 2011.75.

[39] Asanuma Y, Oeser A, Shintani AK, Turner E, Olsen N, Fazio S, Linton MF, Raggi P, Stein CM. Premature coronary-artery atherosclerosis in systemic lupus erythematosus. N Engl J Med. 2003 Dec 18;349(25):2407-15.

[40] Roman MJ, Crow MK, Lockshin MD, Devereux RB, Paget SA, Sammaritano L, Levine DM, Davis A, Salmon JE. Rate and determinants of progression of atherosclerosis in systemic lupus erythematosus. Arthritis Rheum. 2007 Oct;56(10):3412-9.

[41] Roman MJ, Shanker BA, Davis A, Lockshin MD, Sammaritano L, Simantov R, Crow MK, Schwartz JE, Paget SA, Devereux RB, Salmon JE. Prevalence and correlates of accelerated atherosclerosis in systemic lupus erythematosus. N Engl J Med. 2003 Dec 18;349(25):2399-406. Erratum in: N Engl J Med. 2006 Oct 19;355(16):1746.

[42] Esdaile JM, Abrahamowicz M, Grodzicky T, Li Y, Panaritis C, du Berger R, Côte R, Grover SA, Fortin PR, Clarke AE, Senécal JL. Traditional Framingham risk factors fail to fully account for accelerated atherosclerosis in systemic lupus erythematosus. Arthritis Rheum. 2001 Oct;44(10):2331-7.

[43] Kiani AN, Post WS, Magder LS, Petri M. Predictors of progression in atherosclerosis over 2 years in systemic lupus erythematosus. Rheumatology (Oxford). 2011 Nov; 50(11):2071-9. Epub 2011 Aug 28.

[44] Manzi S, Meilahn EN, Rairie JE, Conte CG, Medsger TA Jr, Jansen-McWilliams L, D'Agostino RB, Kuller LH. Age-specific incidence rates of myocardial infarction and angina in women with systemic lupus erythematosus: comparison with the Framingham Study. Am J Epidemiol. 1997 Mar 1;145(5):408-15.

[45] Bengtsson C, Bengtsson A, Costenbader Kh, Jönsen A, Rantapää-Dahlqvist S, Sturfelt G, Nived O.Systemic lupus erythematosus and cardiac risk factors: medical record documentation and patient adherence.Lupus. 2011 Oct;20(10):1057-62. Epub 2011 Jun 15.

[46] Dhar JP, Essenmacher L, Ager J, Chiodo L, Schultz D, Stark A, Schwartz A, Gregoire L, Sokol RJ. Premature cardiovascular aging in women with systemic lupus erythematosus. Presented at the 59th Annual Scientific Meeting of the Society of Gynecological Investigation, San Diego, California, March 2012 and Reproductive Sciences 19 (3 supplement):T-196, 2012.

[47] Chiu CC, Huang CC, Chan WL, Chung CM, Huang PH, Lin SJ, Chen JW, and Leu HB. Increased Risk of Ischemic Stroke in Patients with Systemic Lupus Erythematosus:A Nationwide Population-based Study. Intern Med 51: 17-21, 2012 DOI: 0.2169/internalmedicine.51.6154

[48] Wang IK, Muo CH, Chang YC, Liang CC, Lin SY, Chang CT, Yen TH, Chuang FR, Chen PC, Huang CC, Sung FC. Risks, subtypes, and hospitalization costs of stroke among patients with systemic lupus erythematosus: a retrospective cohort study in Taiwan. J Rheumatol. 2012 Aug;39(8):1611-8. Epub 2012 Jul 1.

[49] Stefanidou S, Benos A, Galanopoulou V, Chatziyannis I, Kanakoudi F, Aslanidis S, Boura P, Sfetsios T, Settas L, Katsounaros M, Papadopoulou D, Giamalis P, Dombros N, Chatzistilianou M, and Garyfallos A. Clinical expression and morbidity of systemic lupus erythematosus during a post-diagnostic 5-year follow-up: a male:female comparison. Lupus (2011) 20, 1090–1094.

[50] Brey RL, Muscal E, and Chapman J. Antiphospholipid antibodies and the brain: A consensus report. Lupus 2011 20: 153.

[51] Hortsman LL, Jy W, Bidot CJ, et al. Antiphospholipid antibodies: paradigm in transition. J Neuroinflammation 2009: 6: 3 From BREY

[52] Aksu K, Donmez A., and Kese, G..Inflammation-Induced Thrombosis: Mechanisms, Disease Associations and Management. Current Pharmaceutical Design, 2012, 18, 1478-1493

[53] Tichelaar YIGV, Kluin-Nelemans HJC, Karina-Meijer K. Infections and inflammatory diseases as risk factors for venous thrombosis. Thromb Haemost 2012; 107: 827–837

[54] Nicolaides AN, Breddin HK, Carpenter P, Coccheri S, Conrad J, De Stefano V, Elkoo-
      fy N, Gerotziafas G, Guermazi S, Haas S, Hull R, Kalodiki E, Kristof V, Michiels JJ,
      Myers K, Pineo G, Prandoni P, Romeo G, Samama MM, Simonian S, Xenophontos S.
      Consensus Statement: Thrombophilia and Venous Thromboembolism. International
      Consensus Statement. Guidelines according to scientific evidence. International
      Angiology 2005; 24: 1-26.

[55] Margetic S, Inflammation and haemostasis. Biochemia Medica 2012;22(1):49–62

[56] Vila LM, Alarcon GS, McGwin G, Bastian HM, Fessler BJ, Reveille JD; LUMINA
      Study Group. Systemic lupus erythematosus in a multiethnic cohort (LUMINA):
      XXIX. Elevation of erythrocyte sedimentation rate is associated with disease activity
      and damage accrural. J Rheumatol 2005; 32: 2150-5.

[57] Pullmann Jr. R, Skerenova M, Lukac J, Hybenova J, Melus V, Kubisz P, Rovensky J,
      Pullman J. Factor V Leiden and Prothrombin G20210A mutations and the risk of
      atherothrombotic events in systemic lupus erythematosus. Clinical and Applied
      Thrombosis/Hemostasis 2004; 10: 233-8.

[58] Oikonomopoulou K, Ricklin D, Ward PA, John D, Lambris JD. Interactions between
      coagulation and complement—their role in Inflammation. Semin Immunopathol.
      2012 January ; 34(1): 151–165. doi:10.1007/s00281-011-0280-x.

[59] Sailer T, Vormittag R, Pabinger I, Vukovich T, Lehr S, Quehenberger P, Panzer S,
      Lechner K, Zoghlami-Rintelen C. Inflammation in patients with lupus anticoagulant
      and implications for thrombosis. J Rheumatol. 2005 Mar;32(3):462-8.

[60] Ames PR, Alves J, Pap AF, Ramos P, Khamashta MA, Hughes GR.Fibrinogen in sys-
      temic lupus erythematosus: more than an acute phase reactant? J Rheumatol. 2000
      May;27(5):1190-5.

[61] Kiraz S, Ertenli I, Benekli M, Haznedaroğlu IC, Calgüneri M, Celik I, Apraş S, Kirazli
      S. Clinical significance of hemostatic markers and thrombomodulin in systemic lu-
      pus erythematosus: evidence for a prothrombotic state. Lupus. 1999;8(9):737-41.

[62] Frieri M. Accelerated atherosclerosis in systemic lupus erythematosus: role of proin-
      flammatory cytokines and therapeutic approaches. Curr Allergy Asthma Rep. 2012
      Feb;12(1):25-32.

[63] Male C, Foulon D, Hoogendoom H, Vegh P, Silverman E, David M, Mitchell L. Pre-
      dictive value of persistent versus transient antiphospholipid subtypes for the risk of
      thrombotic events in pediatric patients with systemic lupus erythematosus. Blood
      2005; 106: 4152-8.

[64] Alfetra A, Vadacca M, Conti L, Galluzo S, Mitterhofer AP, Ferri GM, Del- Porto F,
      Caccavo D, Gandolfo GM, Amoroso A. Thrombosis in systemic lupus erythemato-
      sus: congenital and acquired risk factors. Arthritis and Rheumatism 2005; 53: 452-9.

[65] Onetti L, Villafane S, Menso E, Drenkard C, Gamron S, Barberis G, Onetti CM. Hy-
      perhomocysteinemia as a thrombotic risk factor in patients suffering from systemic

lupus erythematosus and antiphospholipid syndrome. Rev Fac Cien Med Univ Nac Cordoba 2005; 62: 19-23.

[66] Petri M, Roubenoff R, Dallal G, Nadeau MR, Selhub J, Rosenberg IH. Plasma homocysteine as a risk factor for atherothrombotic events in systemic lupus erythematosus. The Lancet 1996; 348: 1120-4.

[67] Bertolaccini M, Mepani K, Sanna G, Hughes GR, Khamashta, MA. Faxtor XII autoantibodies as a novel marker for thrombosis and adverse obstetric history n patients with systemic lupus erythematosus. Ann Rheum Dis 2007; 66:533-6

[68] Bizzaro N, Ghiradelio A, Zampieri S, Iaccarino L, Tozzoli R, Ruffatti A, Villalta D, Tonutti E, Doria A. Anti-thrombotic autoantibodies predict thrombosis in patients with systemic lupus erythematosus: a 15 year longitudinal study. J Thromb Haemost 2007 March 21 Epub ahead of print.

[69] de Laat B, Wu XX, van Lummel M, Derksen RHWM, de Groot PG, Rand JH. Correlation between antiphospholipid antibodies that recognize domain I of β2-glycoprotein 1 and a reduction in the anticoagulant activity of annexin A5. Blood 2007; 109: 1490-4.

[70] Esposito G, Tamby MC, Chanseaud Y, Servettaz A, Guillevin L, Mouthon L. Autoimmunity reviews 2005; 4: 53-60.

[71] Cererholm A, Svenungsson E, Jensen-Urstad K, Trollmo G, Ulfgren AK, Svendenborg J, Fei GZ, Frostegard J. Decreased binding of Annexin V to entothelial cells: a potential mechanism in atherothrombosis of patients with systemic lupus erythematosus. Artheriosclerosis, Thrombosis, and Vascular Biology 2005; 25: 198-203.

[72] Petri M. Epidemiology of the antiphospholipid antibody syndrome. Journal of Autoimmunity 2000; 15: 145-51.

[73] Petri M. Thrombosis and systemic lupus erythematosus: the Hopkins Lupus Cohort perspective. Scand J Rheumatol 1996; 25: 191-3.

[74] Barcat D, Guerin V, Ryman A< Constans J, Vernhes JP, Vergnes C, Bonnet F, Delbrel X, Marlat P, Longy-Boursier M, Conri C. Thrombophilia and thrombosis in systemic lupus erythematosus; a case control study. Ann Rheum Dis 2003; 62: 1016-7.

[75] Mok CC, Tang SSK, To CH, Petri M. Incidence and risk factors of thromboembolism in systemic lupus erythematosus. A comparison of three ethnic groups. Arthritis and Rheumatism 2005; 52: 2774-82.

[76] Clouse MEB, Magder LS, Witter F, Petri M. Early risk factors for pregnancy loss in lupus. Obstetrics & Gynecology 2006; 107: 293-9

[77] Male C, Foulon D, Hoogendoom H, Vegh P, Silverman E, David M, Mitchell L. Predictive value of persistent versus transient antiphospholipid subtypes for the risk of thrombotic events in pediatric patients with systemic lupus erythematosus. Blood 2005; 106: 4152-8.

[78] Alfetra A, Vadacca M, Conti L, Galluzo S, Mitterhofer AP, Ferri GM, Del- Porto F, Caccavo D, Gandolfo GM, Amoroso A. Thrombosis in systemic lupus erythematosus: congenital and acquired risk factors. Arthritis and Rheumatism 2005; 53: 452-9

[79] Chen PP, Wu M, Hahn BH. Some antiphospholipid antibodies bind to various serine proteases in hemostasis and tip the balance toward hypercoagulant states. Lupus 2010 19: 365

[80] Mackworth-Young CG. Antiphospholipid syndrome: multiple mechanisms. Clin Exp Immunol 2004; 136: 393-401.

[81] Mehdi AA, Uthman I, and Khamashta M. Antiphospholipid syndrome: pathogenesis and a window of treatment opportunities in the future. Eur J Clin Invest 2010; 40 (5): 451–464

[82] Adams MJ, Palatinus AA, Harvey AM, and Khalafallah AA. Impaired control of the tissue factor pathway of blood coagulation in systemic lupus erythematosus. Lupus 2011 20: 1474

[83] Tripodi A, deGroot PG, and Pengo V. Antiphospholipid syndrome: laboratory detection,mechanisms of action and treatment. J Intern Med 2011; 270: 110–122.

[84] van Os GMA, Urbanus RT, Aga, C, Meijers JCM, and de Groot PG. Antiphospholipid syndrome:Current insights into laboratory diagnosis and Pathophysiology. Hämostaseologie 2010; 30: 139–143

[85] Matsuura E, Shen L, Matsunami Y, Quan N, Makarova M, Geske FJ, Boisen M, Yasuda S, Kobayashi K, and Lopez LR. Pathophysiology of b2-glycoprotein I in antiphospholipid syndrome. Lupus 2010 19: 379

[86] Devreese KMJ, Standardization of antiphospholipid antibody assays. Where do we stand? Lupus 2012 21: 718

[87] Devreese K, Hoylaerts MF. Challenges in the Diagnosis of the Antiphospholipid Syndrome. Clinical Chemistry 56:6; 930–940 (2010)

[88] RAS Roubey. Risky business: the interpretation, use, and abuse of antiphospholipid antibody tests in clinical practice. Lupus 2010 19: 440

[89] Pengo V, Denas G, Banzato A, Bison E, Bracco A, Visentin MS, Hoxha A, and Ruffatti A. Interpretation of laboratory data and need for reference laboratories. Lupus 2012 21: 732

[90] Bertolaccini ML, Amengual O, Atsumi T, Binder WL, de Laat B, Forastiero R, Kutteh WH, Lambert M, Matsubayashi H, Murthy V, Petri M, Rand JH, Sanmarco M, Tebo AE, and Pierangeli SS. 'Non-criteria' aPL tests: report of a task force and preconference workshop at the 13th International Congress on Antiphospholipid Antibodies, Galveston, TX, USA, April 2010. Lupus 2011 20: 191

[91]   Pierangeli SS, Harris EN. A protocol for determination of anticardiolipin antibodies by ELISA. Nat P rotoc 2008;3:840–8.

[92]   Petri M, Roubenoff R, Dallal G, Nadeau MR, Selhub J, Rosenberg IH. Plasma homocysteine as a risk factor for atherothrombotic events in systemic lupus erythematosus. The Lancet 1996; 348: 1120-4.

[93]   Martínez-Berriotxoa A, Ruiz-Irastorza G, Egurbide MV, Rueda M, Aguirre C. Homocysteine, antiphospholipid antibodies and risk of thrombosis in patients with systemic lupus erythematosus. Lupus. 2004;13(12):927-33.

[94]   Barcat D, Guérin V, Ryman A, Constans J, Vernhes JP, Vergnes C, Bonnet F, Delbrel X, Morlat P, Longy-Boursier M, Conri C. Thrombophilia and thrombosis in systemic lupus erythematosus: a case-control study. Ann Rheum Dis. 2003 Oct;62(10):1016-7

[95]   Vaya A, Calvo J, Alcala C, Mico L, Todol J, Ricart JM. Rheological alterations and thrombotic events in patients with systemic lupus erythematosus. Clinical Hemorhology and Microcirculation: 51; 2012: 51-58

[96]   Kaiser R, Li Y, Chang M, Catanese J, Begovich AB, Brown EE, Edberg JC, McGwin Jr. G, Alarcon GS, Ramsey-Goldman R, Reville JD, Vila LM, Petri MA, Kimberly RP, Kimberly ET and Criswell LA. Genetic Risk Factors for Thrombosis in Systemic Lupus Erythematosus. J Rheumatol 2012;39:1603–10

[97]   Demerci FYK, Dressen AS, Kammerer CM, Barmada MM, Kao AH, Ramsey-Goldman R, Manzi S, Kamboh MI. Functional Polymorphisms of the Coagulation Factor II Gene (F2) and Susceptibility to Systemic Lupus Erythematosus. The Journal of Rheumatology 2011; 38:4

[98]   Terue, R, Perez-Sanchez C, Corral J, Merranz MT, Perez-Andreu V, Salz E, Garcia-Barbera N, Martinez-Martinez I, Roldan V, Vicente V, Lopez-Pedrera C, Martinez C. Identification of miRNAs as potential modulators of tissue factor expression in patients with systemic lupus erythematosus and antiphospholipid syndrome. Journal of Thrombosis and Haemostasis; 9: 1985-1992.

[99]   Bicakcigil M, Tasan DA, Tasdelen N, Mutlu N, and Yavuz S. Role of fibrinolytic parameters and plasminogen activator inhibitor 1 (PAI-1) promoter polymorphism on premature atherosclerosis in SLE patients. Lupus 2011 20: 1063

[100] Gong R, Liu Z, and Li L. Epistatic Effect of Plasminogen Activator Inhibitor 1and Fibrinogen Genes on Risk of Glomerular Microthrombosis in Lupus Nephritis. Arthritis & Rheumatism 2007 56 (5); 1608–1617

[101] Ta'ssies D, Espinosa G, Munoz-Rodriguez FJ, Freire C, Cervera R, Monteagudo J, Maragall S, Escolar G, Ingelmo M, Ordinas A, Font J, and Reverter JC.The 4G/5G polymorphism of the type 1 plasminogen activator inhibitor gene and thrombosis in patients with antiphospholipid syndrome. Arthritis & Rheumatism 2000;43(10):2349–2358

[102] Pereira J, Alfaro G, Goycoolea M, Quiroga T, Ocqueteau M, Massardo L, Perez C, Saez C, Panes O, Matus V, Mezzano D. Circulating platelet –derived microparticles in systemic lupus erythematosus. Association with increased thrombin generation and procoagulant state. Thromb Haemost 2006; 95: 94-9.

[103] Nojima J,Juratsune H, Suehisa E, Kitani T, Iwatani Y, Kanakura Y. Strong correlation between the prevalence of cerebral infarction and the presence of anti-cardiolipin/ beta2-glycoprotein I and antiphosphatidylserine/prothrombin antibodies—Co-existance of these antibodies enhances ADP-induced platelet activation in vitro. Thromb Haemost 2004; 91: 967-76.

[104] Ekdahl KN, Bengtsson AA, Andersson J, Elgue G, Ronnblom L, Sturfelt G, Nilsson B. Thrombotic disease in systemic lupus erythematosus is associated with a maintained systemic platelet activation. Br J Haematol 2004; 125: 74-8.

[105] Levy Y, Shenkman B, Tamarin I, Pauzner R, Shoenfeld Y, Langevitz P, Savion N, Varon D. Increased platelet deposition on extracellular matrix under flow conditions in patients with antiphospholipid syndrome who experience thrombotic events. Arthritis and Rheumatism 2005; 52: 4011-17.

[106] Joseph JE, Harrison P, Mackie IJ, Isenberg DA, Machin SJ. Increased circulating platelet-leukocyte complexes and platelet activation in patients with antiphospholipid syndrome, systemic lupus erythematosus, and rheumatoid arthritis. Br J Haematol 2001; 115: 451-9.

[107] Martinuzzo ME, Maclouf J, Carreras LO, Levy-Toledano S. Antiphospholipid antibodies enhance thrombin-induced platelet activation and thromboxane formation. Thromb Haemost 1993; 70: 667-71.

[108] Vazques-Mellado J, Llorente L, Richaud-Patin Y, Alarcon-Segovia D. Exposure of anionic phospholipids upon platelet activation permits binding of β2 glycoprotein I and through it that of IgG antiphospholipid antibodies: studies in platelets from patients with antiphospholipid syndrome and normal subjects. J Autoimmun 1994; 7: 335-48.

[109] Frenkel EP, Mammen EF. Sticky platelet syndrome and thrombocythemia. Hematol Oncol Clin North Am. 2003 Feb;17(1):63-83.

[110] Mammen EF Sticky platelet syndrome.Semin Thromb Hemost. 1999;25(4):361-5.

[111] Mammen EF, Barnhart MI, Selik NR, Gilroy J, Klepach GL. Sticky platelet syndrome": a congenital platelet abnormality predisposing to thrombosis? Folia Haematol Int Mag Klin Morphol Blutforsch. 1988;115(3):361-5.

[112] Bick RL. Recurrent miscarriage syndrome due to blood coagulation protein/platelet defects: prevalence, treatment and outcome results. DRW Metroplex Recurrent Miscarriage Syndrome Cooperative Group.Clin Appl Thromb Hemost. 2000 Jul;6(3): 115-25.

[113] Weber M, Gerdsen F, Gutensohn K, Schoder V, Eifrig B, Hossfeld DK. Enhanced platelet aggregation with TRAP-6 and collagen in platelet aggregometry in patients with venous thromboembolism.Thromb Res. 2002 Sep 15;107(6):325-8.

[114] Joseph JE, Harrison P, Mackie IJ, Machin SJ.Platelet activation markers and the primary antiphospholipid syndrome (PAPS).Lupus. 1998;7 Suppl 2:S48-51. Review.

[115] Nojima J, Suehisa E, Kuratsune H, Machii T, Koike T, Kitani T, Kanakura Y, Amino N.Platelet activation induced by combined effects of anticardiolipin and lupus anticoagulant IgG antibodies in patients with systemic lupus erythematosus--possible association with thrombotic and thrombocytopenic complications. Thromb Haemost. 1999 Mar;81(3):436-41.

[116] Ekdahl KN, Bengtsson AA, Andersson J, Elgue G, Rönnblom L, Sturfelt G, Nilsson B.Thrombotic disease in systemic lupus erythematosus is associated with a maintained systemic platelet activation.Br J Haematol. 2004 Apr;125(1):74-8.

[117] Urbanus RT, de Laat HB, de Groot PG, Derksen HWM. Prolonged bleeding time and lupus anticoagulant. A second paradox in the anti phospholipid syndrome. Arthritis & Rheumatism 2004; 50: 3605-9

[118] Miyakis S, Lockshin MD, Atsumi D, Branch DW, Brey RL, Cervera R, et al. International consensus statement on an update of the classification criteria for definite antiphospholipid syndrome (APS). J Thromb Haemost 2006;4:295–306.

[119] Bertero MT. Primary prevention in antiphospholipid antibody carriers. Lupus 2012; 21:751

[120] Ruiz-Irastorza G, Cuadrado MJ, Ruiz-Arruza I, et al. Evidence-based recommendations for the prevention and long-term management of thrombosis in antiphospholipid antibody-positive patients: report of a task force at the 13th International Congress on antiphospholipid antibodies. Lupus 2011; 20: 206–218.

[121] Sangle NA, Kristi J, Smock KJ. Antiphospholipid Antibody Syndrome. Arch Pathol Lab Med. 2011;135:1092–1096

[122] Bertsias G, Ioannidis JP, Boletis J, Bombardieri S, Cervera R, Dostal 28 C, et al. EULAR recommendations for the management of systemic lupus erythematosus. Report of a task force of the EULAR Standing Committee for International Clinical Studies Including Therapeutics. Ann Rheum Dis 2008;67:195-205.

[123] Ortel TL. Antiphospholipid syndrome: Laboratory testing and diagnostic strategies. Am. J. Hematol. 2012:87:S75–S81

[124] Tincani A, Andreoli L, Casu C, Cattaneo R, and Meroni P. Antiphospholipid antibody profile: implications for the evaluation and management of patients. Lupus 2010 19: 432

[125]   Branch DW, Khamashta MA. Antiphospholipid syndrome: obstetric diagnosis, management, and controversies. Obstet Gynecol. 2003;101(6):1333–1344.

[126]   Kutteh WH. Antiphospholipid antibody-associated recurrent pregnancy loss: treatment with heparin and low-dose aspirin is superior to low-dose aspirin alone. Am J Obstet Gynecol 1996;174:1584–9.

[127]   Tincani A, Branch W, Levy RA et al. Treatment of pregnant patients with antiphospholipid syndrome.Lupus2003;12:524–9.

[128]   Ruiz-Irastorza G,Khamashta MA. Management of thrombosis in antiphospholipid syndrome and systemic lupus erythematosus in pregnancy. Ann NY Acad Sci 2005; 1051:606–12.

Chapter 6

Thrombophilia in Assisted Reproductive Technology — Place and Needs of Thromboprophylaxis

P. Ivanov, Sl. Tomov, Tsv. Tsvyatkovska,
E. Konova and R. Komsa-Penkova

Additional information is available at the end of the chapter

1. Introduction

Assisted reproductive techniques (ART) have become part of the routine care, with a prevalence ranging from 0.1 to 3.9% of all live born children in Europe and an average of 2% in some parts of the USA [1]. Despite the initial dramatic improvements in success rates and significant increments in ART uptake, the live birth rate resulting from these techniques has recently plateaued. Unfortunately a common non successful termination of ART procedures are due to failure of implantation of high quality graded embryo(s). Implantation failure may recur and three or more in vitro fertilization (IVF) cycles without pregnancy are usually regarded as repeated implantation failures (RIF).

Recently after improving embryo culture media and optimizing controlled ovarian hyperstimulation (COH) protocols, the predominant part of IVF cycles results in embryo transfer (ET) but only about one third [2] of all cycles reach clinically achieved pregnancy. This is evidence that most embryos failed in an early stage of pregnancy establishment. RIF after IVF procedures emphasize the clinical importance of this crucial step in ART and forces efforts to investigate the firm mechanism of implantation and to find approach to increase pregnancy outcome success.

The implantation of the blastocyst into the endometrium in human pregnancy is a very complex corresponding signalling process including specific receptors being expressed on cells surface both on embryo and maternal cells. The specific signalling processes throughout implantation passed in the similar, although not the same algorithm in the spontaneous cycle and after IVF embryo transfer. Plenty of factors have been recognized to affect either success, or failure rate of IVF embryo transfer. Mother side factors include age, parity, hormonal levels before stimulation, antral follicles count, endometrial thickness and quality of transformed endometrium [3, 4]. Embryo grading [5] and place of ET in uterus are other implantation limiting factors. It turns out that not only endometrium, but also extracellular matrix molecules, endothelium and blood circulation factors were involved in remodelling of the endometrium, which is associated with the embryo acceptance process.

A couple of factors [6], having functions in coagulation and fibrinolysis cascades, were found to be connected with the transformation processes in the endometrium during the implantation. In relation with that, the alteration of the function and activity of blood coagulation factors could influence blastocyst acceptance in the endometrium. One proposed cause for implantation failure could be maternal thrombophilias. Thrombophilia was represented as a condition of hypercoagulable state with variety of causes [7] – inherited defects in coagulation factors, anticoagulation and fibrinolysis processes. All these coagulation factors changes result in an increased capacity of blood to form thrombin. The formation of increased thrombin amount, main factor triggering formation of thrombus, is associated with an increased risk of thrombosis development [8]. The study of inherited thrombophilia impact on implantation failure is conducive to IVF procedure because of in vitro embryo selection before transfer. Thus a part of implantation failures due to chromosomal abnormalities [9] of the conceptus have been eliminated as a cause of negative pregnancy outcome.

In the recent twenty years, a number of heritable disorders predisposing to thrombosis have been identified. Except the well-known deficiencies in anticoagulation factors – protein C, S and antithrombin III [10], nowadays, the defects in factor V, factor XIII and factor II of coagulation and polymorphism in plasminogen activator inhibitor (PAI-1) and platelet adhesion proteins [11], have been widely discussed The prevalence of inherited thrombophilic factors in the different populations varies widely from being absent to being found in up to 15% of healthy individuals [12, 13]. In this relation, a discussion of the impact of inherited thrombophilia should be performed only in the range of corresponding population with well-known distribution of factors in health individuals.

Thrombophilic defects have been shown to be associated with an increased risk not only of venous thrombosis but also with fetal loss and gestational complications. Multiple studies [14, 15, 16, 17] have shown that thrombophilias increase the risk of recurrent first- and second-trimester pregnancy losses through placental bed thrombosis. To date, meta-analyses of relatively small case–control studies have demonstrated a small but significant increase (OR 1.5–4.0) in embryonic and fetal loss, abruption, intrauterine growth restriction and preeclampsia in association with inherited thrombophilias [18, 19] Prospective cohort studies have similarly supported a minor contribution of inherited thrombophilias on perinatal outcomes [20, 21].

Maternal risk was also increased with increments in the rates of preeclampsia, gestational diabetes, placenta praevia and the consequent need for Caesarean section. All of these conditions are being increasingly recognized as having their origins in the first trimester with abnormal implantation and trophoblast development being the key pathophysiological processes. Furthermore, several investigators have also studied the relationship between thrombophilias and implantation with conflicting results [22, 23, 24]. An additional confusing fact is that the development of the intervillous space occurs after 10 week of gestation, making it somewhat difficult to explain implantation failure solely with microthrombosis in decidual vessels. Current evidence concerning thrombophilias and recurrent IVF failure remains limited and inconclusive. Therefore, there is need to evaluate the present prominence of the association of inherited thrombophilia factors with IVF failure not only with thrombotic changes during the implantation process, but also to examine the possible influence of the factors on maternal-embryo receptor interaction and the influence on embryo development.

The notion that coagulation disorders may lead to implantation failure has led to the use of anticoagulants, mainly heparin, during assisted reproduction. The role of heparin in assisted conception in women with inherited and acquired thrombophilia has been thought classically to be prevention of thrombosis in relation to implantation and placental development. It is postulated, potentially, a much wider role for heparin in assisted conception due to its ability to interact with a wide variety of proteins, which can alter the physiological processes of implantation and trophoblast development, a process that may be adversely influenced by assisted conception per se. Although the process of implantation is enigmatic, anticoagulant therapy is now being examined as a preventative measure for women with a history of placental-mediated pregnancy complications and many clinics are embarking on the use of low molecular weight heparins (LMWH), again based on biological plausibility rather than evidence of efficacy. Despite the heterogeneity of studies, the results suggest a potential improvement in pregnancy outcomes with anticoagulant therapy.

The approval of the outlined potential of LMWH to alter the molecular processes underpinning successful implantation is urgently required giving the potential for clinical translation to increased pregnancy and live birth rate and a reduction in adverse perinatal outcomes for all women undergoing ART. Important notes discuss the present chapter connected with appropriate time, type and dose of anticoagulant prophylaxis according to patients' type and severity of thrombophilia. This was given after elucidation of the place of inherited thrombo-philic factors in implantation process and type and action of some off-label drugs used in improving ART success.

2. Overview of human embryo implantation stages. Adhesion glycoproteins and coagulation factors in implantation process

In the middle of the eighties it was found that the implantation is not one-stage process in primates [25] and is subdivided in a few separate different steps in which many factors both from the mother and embryo have been involved. Prior to the real implantation and after the shedding of zona pellucida, the embryo is oriented toward the endometrium. This stage of implantation was named apposition. During this process, there is no contact between embryo and endometrial cells. The apposition was followed by an adhesion of the embryo to the endometrial cells surface. This step was time limited and was performed through cell surface receptor communication. In the window of implantation [26] – a short period where it is only possible to realize the implantation process, both endometrial and embryonic cells express adhesion molecules and materialize the adhesion. The adhesion molecules are mainly receptors form the integrin family [27]. Generally, integrins are a group of cell surface adhesion molecules playing role in allowing cell to cell interaction. Within the endometrium, the expression of certain integrins changes during the menstrual cycle [28, 29]. Three integrins, in particular $\alpha v\beta 3$, $\alpha 4\beta 1$ and $\alpha 1\beta 1$, are thought to play a vital role in the implantation. $\alpha v\beta 3$ is the integrin which amount changes most prominently during the implantation window. Heterodimer $\alpha v\beta 3$ consists of two subunits αv and $\beta 3$, which execute different functions. $\beta 3$ subunit is connected with receptor-to-receptor interaction: the subunit recognizes the extracellular matrix ligand osteopontin, which is a protein ligand expressed by the endometrium during the window of implantation. The interaction between integrin $\alpha v\beta 3$ on endometrial and embryonic cell surface with ostepontin actually realize first cell-to-cell contact – embryo adhesion [30]. The expression of the intact heterodimer $\alpha v\beta 3$ is rate-limited by the production of the $\beta 3$ subunit, which is regulated directly by the transcription factors. $\beta 3$ subunit also is a part of other integrins. One of them is $\alpha IIb\beta 3$ integrin, involved in the process of platelet aggregation [31]. One common polymorphism in the gene sequence of $\beta 3$ subunit (1567 T>C) was found to increase the subunit affinity to ligands and could influence the platelet interaction, as well as the adhesion process during implantation.

The last and the most extended and complex process during implantation is the trophoblast invasion within endometrium. The trophoblast invasion requires plenty of up- and down-regulation of many factors both from mother and embryo, which results in degradation of decidua extracellular matrix (ECM) and subsequently endometrium and myometrium vessels invasion. The initial invasion of the throphoblast into the decidua requires the up-regulation of proteases (especially matrix metalloproteinases - MMP) to degrade the ECM. The enzyme activity of migration-behaviour part of cytotrophoblast – extravillous cytotrophoblast (EVT), is controlled by urokinase plasminogen activator (uPA) [32]. uPA is able to activate matrix metalloproteinases (MMPs), produced by EVTs. In vitro studies have shown that after activation by uPA the migrating trophoblast up-regulates MMP2 [33], MMP3, MMP9 [34] and cathepsins [35]. Plasminogen activator inhibitor-1 (PAI-1) is a primary uPA regulator that inhibits uPA by forming a covalent complex, thus controlling the thrombotic/fibrinolytic process [36]. In addition, through its binding to the ECM, PAI-1 regulates cell adhesion and migration by interfering with the binding between cellular integrins or uPA receptor (uPAR) and vitronectin. A 2675 4G/5G sequence polymorphism in the PAI-1 gene promoter has been correlated with increased levels of plasma PAI-1 [37]. The carrier status for 4G4G phenotype results in higher activity than the 5G allele, because in addition to the binding site for the transcriptional activator, the latter also contains a binding site for a transcriptional repressor. In the presence of 4G allele and the absence of bound repressor, the basal level of PAI-1 transcription is increased [38]. The 4G allele of PAI-1 has been recently linked to venous thromboembolism [39] and coronary disease [37], however relation with recurrent pregnancy loss and implantation failure is under discussion.

After the initial invasion into decidua, EVT gains endometrial vessels and breaches their wall allowing first contact of embryo cells with maternal blood [40]. During this deep invasion step, EVT opened and remodelled spiral arteries and arterioles to produce high-conductance vessels, necessary for the further developing fetus. The haemostasis into decidua during vessel invasion was ensured by up-regulation of tissue factor (TF) and activation of extrinsic coagulation cascade, and simultaneously increased PAI-1 activity [41]. The result of increased TF activity is generation of thrombin. In cases of increased thrombin production, such as in inherited thrombophilias conditions, the decidual cells produced anti-angiogenic soluble fms-like tyrosine kinase-1 factor (sFlt-1), which inhibits enzymes related with EVT invasion [41]. Insufficient shallow invasion of ECT into decidua results in incomplete vascular transformation and underperfused embryonic cells, which could lead to early pregnancy loss. Inherited changes in coagulation factors increased the amount of plasma and local thrombin. The most discussed are Factor V Leiden and 20210 G>A substitution in prothormbin gene. The prothrombin (FII) mutation involves guanine-to-adenine transition at nucleotide position in the 3'-untranslated region of the prothrombin gene. The mutation 20210 G>A is associated with both increased plasma concentration of prothrombin, and an increased risk of thrombosis [42]. Factor V Leiden (FVL) represents an altered Factor V (FV) of coagulation proteins, due to substitution of adenine for guanine at nucleotide position 1691 (1691 G>A) in exon 10 of the factor's gene. As a result of the mutation, circulating half time of life of FV is increased dramatically. This has been represented with permanently increased risk for blood clotting formation. This two inherited thrombophilic factors have had still debatable role in increasing the risk for late, as well as early recurrent pregnancy loss.

In the preimplantation period and during the decidual invasion of EVT, simultaneous cell division processes have passed in the embryo. Cell division and differentiation have been connected with continuous changes (activation and inactivation) in gene activity. One fundamental process to regulation of mammalian gene activity is methylation status of the genome [43]. The gene methylation is critical precisely to early embryonic development [44]. Methylation of DNA parts, responsible for gene activity, was realized by donor chemical compounds, such as S-adenosylmethionine (SAM). Methyl groups, passed from folic acid through a series of enzymes, contribute to the production of SAM. As such, folic acid is indispensable for embryonic development [45]. An enzyme critical to the folic acid pathway is methylenetetrahydrofolate reductase (MTHFR). Deficiencies of folic acid or defects in MTHFR have demonstrated DNA hypomethylation and abnormal biochemical and phenotypic changes in cell development and interaction [46, 47].

Most common MTHFR inherited gene changes are 677 C>T 1298 A>C single-nucleotide polymorphisms (SNPs) [48]. Homozygous variant for 677 C>T (genotype TT) creates a thermolabile enzyme with only 30% of wild-type activity. The decreasing of MTHFR activity reduces the amount of SAM and thus methylation processes. Low MTHFR activity causes enzyme block in methionine metabolism and leads to increased homocystein (Hcy) in blood plasma. Concentration of Hcy more than 15 µmoll/ml was found to be related with increased thrombosis development, due to endothelial injure and coagulation cascade activation. The increased plasma Hcy and 677 C>T polymorphism was discussed as a risk factor for arterial and venous thrombosis development. The impact on early pregnancy loss and implantation failure is still disputed point although its role in fertility has not been extensively studied [49, 50, 51]. Another SNP 1298 A>C in MTHFR affects the SAM regulatory domain and has ~60% of wild-type activity [52, 53]. The effect of 1298 A>C on MTHFR and thus on SAM metabolism is not so pronounced as the effect of 677 C>T, and have been discussed as an additional risk factor in presence of both polymorphisms simultaneously.

3. Diverse influence of thrombophilic factors on implantation and risk for RIF

3.1. MTHFR polymorphisms and embryo development

Recent studies try to establish a connection between folic acid metabolism, preimplantation and implantation embryo development. It was shown that folic acid is present in the follicular fluid. Its supplementation decreases serum and follicular fluid homocysteine levels and is associated with better quality and more mature oocytes used in IVF procedures [54]. During maturation oocytes express receptors for folic acid transport protein [55]. This finding enforces the idea for the crucial role of folate and folate metabolism in the regulation of gene expression through methylation and demethylation of regulatory parts of the genes using SAM. By hystopathological investigation some authors have found defective chorionic villous vascularization [56], as well as significantly smaller median area, perimeter and diameter per chorionic vascular element [57] in women with elevated total homocystein levels. Fluctuating data for the prevalence of MTHFR polymorphism in women with repeated IVF failure was presented supporting these hypotheses. Dobson et al. [50] investigated maternal and paternal carrier status for 677 C>T and 1298 A>C in MTHFR in 197 couples, who underwent IVF procedure. They do not found significant impact of both SNPs, although in women with TT genotype decreased pregnancy rate compared with CT and CC genotype was established (33.3% compared with 47.7% and 47.9%). The authors do not exclude any other additional confounding factors concerning IVF failure, such as hyperhomocysteinemia due to alimentary factors or immunological and/or additional thrombophilic factors. Many other authors establish fluctuating prevalence of TT genotype among women failed to conceive after IVF/ICSI: Qublan et al. [24] found 22.2% prevalence of TT genotype. They established this polymorphism as the most common SNP among women with IVF implantation failure. Before that Martinelli et al. [58] found 19% prevalence of TT genotype evaluating 162 women with failed IVF/ICSI treatment. Moreover, Azem et al. [59] who investigated 45 women with a history of four or more failed IVF cycles reported an incidence of 17.8%.

The discrepancy between the reported prevalence could be related with the number of failed IVF cycles [60] in patient groups, as well as with the selection criteria for the control group of women. The isolated impact assessment of MTHFR SNPs depends on a variable number of other investigated thrombophilic factors [22, 23], included in any other study. The ethnic variability of polymorphisms should be also considered. An important obscured factor for difficulties in proper evaluation of MTHFR polymorphism impact is the wide spread prophylactic prenatal vitamins taking containing high dose folic acid. Alimentary intake of folic acid masks the suggested roles of MTHFR genotypes on IVF failure. In relation with that a ten-time increased dose of folic acid supplementation [61, 62,63] was recommended for women undergoing IVF.

3.2. FII 20210 G>A: Thrombin generation influence on cytotrophoblast invasion

Normal implantation is associated with thrombin-induced fibrin deposition in the absence of overt bleeding [64]. The excess of fibrin deposition in forming intervillous spaces could have negative effect on the implantation process. The serine protease thrombin is a key element in fibrin accumulation [23]. In presence of increased amount of thrombin the decidual cells produce anti-angiogenic soluble fms-like tyrosine kinase-1 factor, which inhibits enzymes related with EVT proliferation [41]. Thus in early pregnancy, thrombin may act as an autocrine/ paracrine enhancer of sFlt-1 expression on the decidual cells to promote implantation failure by interfering with local vascular transformation [64]. The prothrombin role on implantation was supported by experimental data for reduced infertility due to increased topical concentration of thrombin in both fallopian tubes, although the mechanism of action of locally administrated thrombin is undefined [65]. The possible impact of FII 20210 G>A on the implantation failure is also supported by the found distinct prevalence of FII 20210 G>A and FVL on early pregnancy loss [66]. In recurrent pregnancy loss before 10 week of gestation was established a more pronounced prevalence of 20210 G>A mutation compared with FVL. The slight increase of APC (natural inhibitor of FV) at early pregnancy could explain normal level of FV activity during the embryonic period (5 to 10 week of gestation) [67]. Indirectly, this finding could be referred to a high prevalence of 20210 G>A mutation in IVF failure. Some studies fail to find relation between 20210 G>A mutation and implantation failure. Others establish weak [23] or strong [24] correlation between 20210 G>A and unsuccessful IVF attempts. The prevalence of FII 20210 G>A in Caucasian is between 1 and 3% and thus the low occurrence enforces larger study arrangement to evaluate the factor's impact on implantation.

3.3. Advantages and disadvantages of FVL during implantation

One of the first and frequently discussed studies concerning IVF failure and presence of inherited thrombophilia is published by Grandone at al. [68]. The study includes a small number of women with more than 3 failed IVF attempts (n=18) compared with 216 women with at least one successful terminated pregnancy. The authors reported significantly higher occurrence of FVL and FII 20210 G>A in patients comparing with controls, although the frequency of FVL in health subjects was found relatively low (1.9%) (common occurrence in Caucasians between 7 and 10% [13]). These authors included in the patients' group women with pregnancy loss, which moreover embarrassed the evaluation of the impact of thrombophilic factors on implantation process. After this report, series of consequent papers discussed the influence of thrombophilia on implantation process, especially after IVF procedure. Some studies found [23, 24] but others not [58, 69] a relation of FVL and FII 20210 G>A with implantation failure. The conflicting results show the necessity of large and specific inclusion criteria fulfilling studies to detect the real connection between the presence of increased thrombin generating factors and implantation outcomes. Interesting diverse outcomes for the prevalence were found by some authors: a part of them established a relatively lower prevalence of FVL in women with IVF implantation failure compared with controls [60]; others reported an increased implantation success after the first IVF attempt in FVL carriers. On this basis the hypothesis for positive effect of thrombin deposition during trophoblastic invasion was established. This selective advantage of FVL carriers on implantation was described for the first time by Gopel et al. [70], who found 90% successful implantation rate after first IVF attempt in FVL carriers comparing to 49% rate in non-carriers. It should be known that the authors included both mother and fetus positive FVL genotype. This stand referred to another discussion concerning the significance of paternal [71] and fetal thrombophilia for early pregnancy development [72]. Similar results show Martinelli et al. [58] reporting 86% pregnancy rate after first IVF attempt in FVL and FII 20210 G>A carriers compared to 68% pregnancy rate in non-carriers (non-significant difference). Although not all authors [72] share the proposition, FVL could improve implantation rate in IVF and spontaneous cycles. The increased implantation rate in FVL carriers could have been balanced by abortions or miscarriages later in pregnancy. The discussions for evolutional advantages and disadvantages of FVL still remain, probably because there should be some unknown benefits, or the mutation would have been eradicated from population.

3.4. PAI-1 4G/5G: Hypofibrinolysis and impaired deep cytotrophoblast invasion

During implantation, an accurate balance of coagulation, fibrin deposition and fibrinolysis is mandatory for trophoblastic invasion. Accumulation of fibrin forces conversion of plasminogen to plasmin, thus stimulating the process of fibrinolysis. Fibrinolysis is important for modulation of the extracellular matrix mediated by the plasminogen activation system. Plasminogen activation facilitates cell migration through targeted proteolysis and local dissolution of the basement membrane [73] So extended fibrinolysis is crucial for implantation process. Inhibition of fibrinolysis after increased activity of plasminogen activator inhibitors such as PAI-1 could impair proper deep trophoblastic invasion. High PAI-1 activity, particularly due to inherited changes in PAI-1 gene expression, is associated with inhibition of the conversion of plasminogen to plasmin and subsequent hypofibrinolysis. Hypofibrinolysis as a result of the 4G allele (especially genotype 4G/4G) of the PAI-1 gene appears to be a possible risk factor for implantation failure by limiting trophoblastic invasion [74].

A limited number of papers report for a possible negative impact of 4G/4G genotype on impaired implantation process. Coulam et al. [23], who investigated 42 women with implantation failure, found a significantly higher prevalence of 4G/4G genotype in patients compared with controls (respectively 38% and 10%). They also found distinct higher occurrence of 4G allele in patients vs. controls (74% and 20%, p=0.007). Goodman et al. [22] also found higher but not significant prevalence of 4G/4G genotype in 73 controls and 70 women experiencing implantation failure (26% vs. 36%). Some others [75] found similar high prevalence of polymorphisms but they also included women with early pregnancy loss in the study group. The impact of 4G/5G polymorphism frequently was evaluated in the context of multigenetic carrier status [23].

3.5. PL A1/A2 in integrin beta 3 platelet activity and adhesion properties of endometrium

To the best of recently knowledge, a few observations have been published on the possible association between the platelet integrin polymorphisms and recurrent pregnancy loss development. The hypothesis for the connection between PL A1/A2 of GP IIb/IIIa and increased risk of pregnancy loss has been based on the supposition that impairment of platelet function is related with disturbance in uteroplacental vascular system. Increased platelet aggregation, as a result of the presence of allele A2 could establish prothrombotic conditions and increase thrombus formation in intervillous space, leading to poor fetal outcome.

Some recent studies find association between beta 3 integrin and recurrent pregnancy loss [76] In our pilot study [60] of 67 women with primary sterility and 96 healthy control subjects, we found a significantly higher prevalence of PL A1/A2 in women with implantation failure after assisted reproduction technology (ART) in comparison with controls (OR: 2.6, 95% CI: 1.1-6.3, p=0.033). These data suggest that the carriers of PL A1/A2 are at higher risk of implantation failure and do not have successful ART outcome. In a separate study [77] we have found more pronounce prevalence of PL A1/A2 in women with RPL before 10 week of gestation compared with carriers status in women with late pregnancy loss (after 10 week of gestation) (41.8% vs 29.3%, OR 1.73; 95% CI 0.93 - 3.21, p=0.084). Compared patients' groups were not FVL and/or FII 20210 G>A carriers. This finding emphasizes the more probable PL A1/A2 influence on early than late pregnancy loss. The impact of increased platelet activity on implantation process is particularly embarrassed, because investigated polymorphism A1/A2 concerns beta3 subunits of platelet integrin alphaIIb/beta3, which is also part of integrin $\alpha v\beta 3$, related with embryo adhesion to endometrium [78]. An in vitro investigation has found that changes in the peptide structure of beta3 subunit have had influence on the receptor activity to its ligands - osteopontin and vitronectin [31]. Sajid et al. [31] established that cell lines which expressed alphaV/beta3 receptor with PL A1/A2 had an enhanced haptotactic migratory response to vitronectin and osteopontin. As the initiation of fetus adhesion to the endometrium has been connected mainly with the activity of integrin alphaV/beta3, polymorphism A1/A2 could play a significant role not only in platelet aggregation, but also in adhesion and endometrium to embryo interaction during implantation.

The influence of thrombophilic genetic factors in pregnancy outcome after assisted reproduction is connected with modification of endometrium adhesion properties and effect on trophoblastic invasion ability. Independent significance of thrombophilia is hard to evaluate because of assembled information for many other recently discussed IVF failure risk factors which are outside the thrombophilic group factors. Apoptosis and cell arrest tumor suppressor factor p53 [79], inducing angiogenesis vascular endothelial growth factor (VEGF) [80] or Leukemia inhibitory factor (LIF) [81] are a part of these agents. These factors should be considered in the impact of thrombophilic factors discussion because the recent approach in consultation after IVF failure investigations is to identify the combination of defects [80] instead of one factor that will lead to implantation failure. Moreover, the fetal role in thrombophilia should also be discussed because of established positive polymorphism carrier status in placental tissue [82]. This finding necessarily includes a role of the father's genetic pattern in pregnancy destiny. Nevertheless the beginning of adequate trophoblastic invasion is tightly regulated by thrombophilic genetic factors expression. Hence, increased activity of one or more thrombogenic agents could modify implantation process. To improve pregnancy outcome after assisted reproduction the type, dose and beginning of effective treatment for imbalances in expression of haemostatic proteins at the time of implantation needs to be established.

4. LMWH action in implantation beyond anticoagulant effects

The role of heparin in assisted conception in improving outcomes in women with inherited or acquired thrombophilia has been thought classically to be prevention of thrombosis in relation to implantation and placental development. But there is, potentially, a much wider role for heparin in assisted conception due to its ability to interact with a wide variety of proteins which have been involved in implantation process [83,84]. Heparin's influence on the physiological processes of implantation and trophoblast development, due to interaction with this growth factors and adhesion molecules responsible for embryo adhesion and invasion could influence the assisted conception entirely. Several lines of evidence from in vivo and in vitro studies suggest a beneficial effect of heparin on embryo implantation through interactions with several adhesion molecules, growth factors, cytokines and enzymes such as matrix metalloproteinases [83]. This finding clarified non-related with coagulation beneficial effect of heparins upon implantation processes.

L-Selectin. Interaction between adhesion molecules on throphoblast and endometrial cells is mediated by lectins, termed selectins. Three different selectins have been identified: P-, E- and L-selectin - which recognize and bind to crucial carbohydrate determinants on selectin ligands. On the blastocyst side, strong L-selectin staining has been observed over the entire embryo surface corresponding to oligosaccharide-based ligands on the maternal side which are up-regulated during the window of implantation [85]. The selectin adhesion system may therefore constitute an initial step in the implantation process. Heparin may have negative effect on selectin-mediated cell adhesion. The inhibitory effect is molecular weight dependent: Tinza-parin, which is known to have about 22–36% fragments greater than 8 kDA, also significantly impaired L-selectin binding, while, enoxaparin with 0–18% fragments > 8 kDa did not impact on L-selectin expression [86] Therefore, care with the choice of LMWH depending form molecular weight would be required, as the use of UFH or a LMWH with a high contribution of large fragments could impair selectin expression and implantation.

Glycoproteins. E-cadherin, a glycoprotein connected with cell-to-cell adhesion is expressed by a variety of tissues including endometrium. The suppression of E-cadherin expression is associated with disruption of cell-to-cell adhesion and acquisition of invasive growth [87]. E-cadherin is up-regulated by estradiol via the estrogen receptor beta and down-regulated by progesterone [88]. Down regulation by increased progesterone levels during luteal phase of cycle facilitated throphoblast invasion. Heparins, particularly enoxaparin have been shown to down-regulate decidual E-cadherin expression [89], thereby potentially explaining the observations that LMWH can promote extravillous trophoblast differentiation

4.1. Local growth factors

Heparin-binding (HB) epidermal growth factor (EGF)-like growth factor functions as a mitogen and is potent survival factor during stress [90]. It has been shown that cells expressing the transmembrane form of HB-EGF adhere to human blastocysts and HB-EGF acts like a potent growth factor for enhancing embryo development to blastocyst and mediation of embryo hatching [91]. Separately, in cell culture was found enhanced differentiation and invasive activity of first trimester trophoblast in presence of HB-EGF. HB-EGF activation is heparins- dependable and therefore, LMWH may potentiate HB-EGF function [92].

Insulin-like growth factors I (IGF-I) and II (IGF-II) are potent mitogenic and differentiation-promoting growth factors and are also implicated in implantation and fetal development [93]. Importantly, they have their activity modulated by glucoseaminoglycans, in particular hepains [94]. Heparin and LMWH increase free IGF-I in a dose-dependent manner and so facilitated implantation [95].

4.2. Cytokines

Transforming growth factors (TGF) β1 to 3 are expressed both in endometrial and trophoblast cells, and have been shown to inhibit trophoblast proliferation and invasion [96]. LMWH inhibits TGF-b1 expression, attenuates collagen and fibronectin deposition and assists throphoblast invasion [97].

Leukaemia inhibitory factor (LIF), is known to regulate differentiation, proliferation and survival of various cells in the embryo as well as in the adult. It also has been found to enhance the blastocyst formation and hatching [98]. To date, no studies have examined the interaction of LIF and heparin, although the given interactions of HB-EGF and TGF-b1 with heparin, potential up-regulation of LIF expression is feasible with experimental analysis urgently required [85].

The presence of **Interleukin-1 (IL-1)**, a pro-inflammatory cytokine in the site of implantation increases endometrial epithelial cell β3 integrin expression with an improved blastocyst adhesion [99]. The effect of LMWH on trophoblast or blastocyst IL-1 expression has not been examined but the found increase of IL-1 expression in activated leukocytes again raising the possibility that modulation of integrin expression may be possible [100].

Interleukin-11 (IL-11) is another pleiotropic cytokine which functions as a hematopoietic growth factor and immunoregulator exhibiting anti-inflammatory effects by regulating immune effector cell function but has additional positive roles in decidualization [101]. The augmentation of IL-11 signalling and induction by heparin may prove to be beneficial both in terms of implantation and placental development [102].

IL-6 in addition to its roles as adipokine, which regulates the acute phase response and haematopoesis, is also implicated in reproduction [103]. The effect of heparin on endometrial IL-6 production is not known but LMWH stimulates IL-6 production by peripheral blood and also enoxaparin had identical effects to recombinant IL-6 in reducing embryonic absorption in a pro-abortive murine model [104].

Granulocyte-macrophage colony-stimulating factor (GM-CSF) stimulates proliferation and differentiation of myeloid precursors into several cell types, but it is also an important determinant of pregnancy outcome: the factor actions as an immune-regulatory agent contributing to maternal immune tolerance of the fetal–placental tissues, and as a trophic growth and viability factor in preimplantation embryo development and regulation of placental morphogenesis [105]. LMWH is also capable of binding to GM-CSF [106]. Again although direct evidence for heparin is lacking, a positive effect on this pathway is possible.

Matrix metalloproteinases (MMPs). MMPs are a family of 22 endopeptidases capable of degrading all components of the ECM and are important mediators of cell behaviour including cell–matrix and cell–cell interactions. In vitro studies suggest that successful implantation and placentation result from the balance between secretion of MMPs from the trophoblast and their inhibition by their natural antagonist tissue inhibitors [107]. The gene knockout studies in mice suggest that MMP-9 is critical for implantation [108]. MMP-9 is known to degrade collagen IV, the main component of the basement membrane, and in conjunction with MMP-2 may enable the invasion of trophoblast cells through the decidua and into the maternal vasculature [109]. Although divergent effects of heparin on MMPs have been observed, LMWH in therapeutic doses has been shown to induce trophoblast MMP-2 and MMP-9 transcription and protein expression. Therefore, LMWH appears capable of improving the invasive capacity of trophoblast cells by regulating MMP degradative capacity [110].

5. Dose and initiation of LMWH therapy in ART according recognized thrombophilic mutations

5.1. Needs of anticoagulant therapy

No guideline suggests a type of pharmacological non-hormonal support for women who have experienced several ART failures with or without thrombophilic factors presence. The possibility that implantation failure depends on hypercoagulability state cannot be ruled out because of a relatively rare investigation of embryo and male partner thrombophilic status. But in IVF/ICSI procedures where embryo aneuploidy, thyroid autoimmunity [111] and other immunological factors [112] are eliminated, and thus high grade embryos are transferred in highly receptive endometrium, therefore inherited thrombophilia could constitute as a main etiologic reason in implantation failure. Also insufficient number randomized studies explore the needs of anticoagulant therapy in RIF and thrombophilia.

The first and last till July 2012 placebo-controlled, randomized trial to evaluate the efficacy of thromboprophylaxis using enoxaparin 40 mg/day in a cohort of 83 women with a history of three or more previous IVF failures, who had at least one thrombophilic defect, was published [113]. Patients who received LMWH for thromboprophylaxis had a significant increase implantation and pregnancy rates compared with the placebo controls (20.9 vs 6.1% and 31 vs 9.6%, respectively; $p < 0.001$ and $p < 0.05$, respectively). A significant increase in the live birth rate was observed in the heparin-treated group compared with placebo (23.8 vs 2.4%, respectively; p <0.01). This study was criticized for its "methodological weakness" and for heparin being used prior to demonstration of its efficacy in carefully designed randomized controlled clinical trials [114]. Disadvantages of this study are the availability in the study group of patients with acquired thrombophilic disorders such as lupus anticoagulant and anticardiolipin antibodies (ACL) which impedes inherited thrombophilia impact evaluation. A weakness is connected also with the insufficient patients' number and not symmetrical appearance of inherited thrombophilic factors among LMWH – treated and non-treated groups.

Some other investigators found a positive impact of LMWH application in women with RIF: Urman et al. [115] found in a cohort of 150 women with two or more failed assisted reproduction treatment cycles, who were randomly assigned to receive 1 mg/kg/day of LMWH or no treatment from oocyte retrieval to 12th week, implantation rates 24.5 and 19.8% in the LMWH and control groups, respectively (p = 0.33), and live births 34.7 versus 26.7%, respectively (p = 0.29). These authors tendentiously excluded from investigation groups women with inherited thrombophilia with intention to avoid possible thrombotic events during implantation process as a result of thrombophilic factors presence.

An interesting study present Lodigiani et al. [116] who introduce LMWH therapy during the time of controlled ovarian hyperstimulation and discontinued on the day of β-human chorionic gonadotrophin application. The authors found an improved outcome of ART in thrombophilic women used 40 mg enoxaparin daily compared with a control group without LMWH (25% vs 13.5% pregnancy rate, p-ns). This study indirectly proved the needs for anticoagulant prophylaxis in thrombophilia presence.

In spite the lack of large randomized trials, an increasing number of clinics embark the use of LMWH prophylaxis in RIF, particular in inherited thrombophilia cases. American College of Chest Physicians (ACCP) Evidence-Based Clinical Practice Guidelines (9th edition, 2012) [117] do not recommend the routine use of LMWH in women with pregnancy complications and inherited thrombophilia, except for the cases of pregnancy after IVF with severe ovarian hyperstimulation syndrome (OHSS) where guidelines recommend a 3 months prophylaxis. A suggestion for the use of prophylactic or intermediate dose LMWH was done only for women carriers of FVL or FII 20120 G>A in homozygous variant who have a family history for venous thromboembolism (VTE). For pregnant women with all other thrombophilias, a close follows up of pregnancy without routine LWMH application has been recommended. The next large number investigation will display the proper place of heparins in implantation failure escape. Until then LMWH prophylaxis should be undertaken with caution, knowing the possible side effects of therapy according to long-term daily treatment. Recommendations for close fallow-up of women with LMWH application was given to avoid bleeding, skin reactions, and heparin-induced thrombocytopenia [118]. Osteoporosis and osteoporotic fractures development was reported only in women with therapeutic dose of LMWH, who have taken more than 30 weeks during pregnancy [119]. All advantages and disadvantages of LMWH prophylaxis should be explicated to women treated with heparins.

5.2. Beginning of LMWH prophylaxis

No consensus concerning initiation of anticoagulant therapy in IVF cycle performance was established. Some authors start the intervention at 6 weeks of gestation following the confirmation of a viable pregnancy and using postulates for early stage of placenta development [120]. As was mentioned, another guideline [116] introduces LMWH therapy during the time of controlled ovarian hyperstimulation, which found improved pregnancy outcome after ART in women with thrombophilic mutations. If it estimates, according founded LMWH action during implantation period, the prophylaxis recommended beginning should be later than embryo transfer day [83, 84].

5.3. Dose regiment of LMWH

When it was referred to VTE events in non-pregnant populations, weight-based LMWH dosage regimens provide effective treatment of acute VTE without the need to monitor anti-Xa levels. In pregnancy, the volume of distribution and renal clearance increases, leading to a lower peak and shorter duration of anti-Xa activity, but with continued use the anti-Xa activity can become prolonged [121] Therapeutic doses after ART may be indicated during pregnancy in women who present with acute VTE, those at high risk of recurrent thromboembolism and women with major cardiac disease at risk of arterial embolism [122]. The therapeutic dose is 1 mg/ kg enoxaparin twice daily. The dose was based on their weight at presentation, rounded to the nearest 10 kg, and was not adjusted as the woman's weight increased during pregnancy. In other cases a prophylactic dose of enoxaparin, 40 mg once daily was recommended: in women with recurrent pregnancy loss with no history of VTE Brenner et al. [123] did not found advantigie to increase enoxaparin from 40 mg/day to 80 mg/day (40 mg twice daily). They found similarly effective and safe the both dose regiments with a live birth of 84% and 78% in the enoxaparin 40 mg/day and 80 mg/day groups, respectively.

5.4. Duration and discontinuation of LMWH therapy

A part of authors discontinued LMWH therapy after the end of 3rd lunar month or in the end of controlled ovarian hyperstimulation [116]. ACCP Guideline recommends discontinuation of LMWH at least 24 h prior to induction of labor or cesarean section (or expected time of neuraxial anesthesia) rather than continuing LMWH until the time of delivery.

5.5. Monitoring of LMWH

Platelet blood count measure was recommended after the start of LMWH prophylaxis to avoid possible complication connected with heparin induced thrombocytopenia (HIT). A poor correlation was found with LMWH use and anti-Xa levels monitoring. Althogh that in prophylactic dose of enoxaparin range of 0.2 to 0.4 U/mL of anti-Xa activity was recommended. When therapeutic dose LMWH was used range of 0.77 to 0.86 U/mL was suggested [124].

Recently a new marker was introduce in monitoring of thrombosis risk patients. Platelet-leukocyte aggregates (PLA) are heterotypic cell complexes. The interaction between platelets and leukocytes manipulates their function in the processes of hemostasis and inflammation [125]. The circulating PLA are a more sensitive marker of in vivo platelet activation than platelet surface P-selectin. PLA could be use as indirect gauge for LMWH therapy in high risk pregnancy complicated in inherited thrombophilia factors [126] because both women with combination of prothrombotic factors and women with single thrombophilic factor showed increased levels of whole blood PLA compared with control group [126].

6. Place of aspirin in RIF – Combined therapy with LMWH

As have been supposed, one of the causes of RIF may be found in impaired uterine perfusion [127]. It has been suggested that Acetylsalicylic acid (low dose aspirin <100 mg/d) may increase the uterine blood flow by inhibiting platelet aggregation and reducing vasoconstriction, possibly leading to a more favourable endometrium for embryo implantation [128]. Aspirin may also suppress the negative effects of prostaglandins on the implantation, such as the induction of uterine contractions or an inflammatory response [129]. Furthermore, aspirin improves the chance of a live birth in women with antiphospholipid syndrome with a history of recurrent miscarriage [130], although newer studies show that it is not effective in women with unexplained recurrent miscarriage [120]. Whereas some studies could not demonstrate any benefit in IVF outcome [131, 132], others reported an increase in pregnancy rate, sometimes with even statistically significant impact [133, 134, 135]. The aspirin influence on IVF outcome and in particular, the action connected with inherited thrombophilia, again is not eluciadated, although Zhao et al. [81] found increased alphaV/beta3 integrin expression in the uterine endometrium in aspirin presence. Speculating from the above finding the polymorphism A1/A2 in beta3 subunits of integrin alphaV/beta3 could be related with impared embryo adhesion but this should be confirmed in future studies. If genotypes A1/A2 and A2/A2 of PL A1/A2 are associated with enhanced platelet thrombogenicity and so with increased risk of implantation failure, an inclusion of prophylactic antiaggregant therapy [136] to prevent poor pregnancy outcome should be considered. Later on, the detecting of the genotype for PL A1/A2 could be important, because of the raised data for acetylsalicylic acid and other antiplatelet agents' resistance [137, 138] in the presence of A2 allele.

Another important gap in the literature was the question when to start and when to stop aspirin and how long should aspirin be given. Usually authors start aspirin just after pregnancy establishment, continue throughout pregnancy and cease 3 weeks before the delivery [139]. Others begin therapy along with the initiation of controlled ovarian hyperstimulation.

In conclusion, in a recent systematic review [140] the authors' conclude that the use of low-dose aspirin for women undergoing IVF could not be recommended due to lack of adequate trial data. Only for women who fulfill the laboratory criteria for antiphopsholipid antibody (APLA) syndrome and meet the clinical APLA criteria based on a history of three or more pregnancy losses, ACCP recommends [117] antepartum administration of low-dose aspirin, 75 to 100 mg/d combined with prophylactic dose LMWH.

7. Metformin, thrombophilia and pregnancy outcome after IVF

Metformin, an oral biguanide insulin-sensitizing agent, acts by inhibiting hepatic glucose production without hypoglycaemia because it does not increase the insulin secretion [141]. This drug enhances the effects of insulin on glucose uptake in skeletal muscles and adipocytes, decreases intestinal absorption of glucose and leads to lowering androgen production in PCO patients [142]. Widely it is known that decreased androgen production after using metformin improves ovulation as well as pregnancy outcome in women with polycystic ovaries [143]. Insulin has a direct effect on ovarian steroidogenesis by the stimulation of androgen production by the thecal cells. Hyperinsulinaemia can inhibit the insulin-like growth factor-1 (IGF-1)-binding protein production by the liver with a subsequent increase in IGF-1. This IGF-1 in conjunction with LH could stimulate ovarian thecal cell androgen production. So, decreasing insulin resistance by metformin recovers menstrual cycle, ovulation and increased pregnancy rate in PCOS. Independently, metformin has a direct inhibitory effect on androstenedione production in human ovarian thecal-like androgen-producing tumour cells [144]. These findings could explain the mechanism for the decrease in androgen levels with the use of metformin. Along with the androgen-decreasing action, metformin was found to reduce plasma plasminogen activator inhibitor-1 (PAI-1) concentration in both diabetic and non-diabetic obese subjects. In vitro studies found dose-dependently decreased PAI-1 production under both basal and interleukin-1 beta-stimulated conditions after metformin application [145]. A large cohort study of PCOS patients has found a relation between the increased prevalence of 4G allele of PAI-1 4G/5G polymorphism and elevated PAI-1 levels [46]. The correlation between the reduction in the plasma insulin and PAI-1 levels after treatment with metformin in early pregnancy, suggests an early initiation of this therapy in COH-IVF cycles. This approach should be considered especially in PCO patients with insulin resistance as well as in patients carriers of 4G allele (homo- and heterozygous state).

If further studies support the reduction of miscarriage rate by metformin, the latter will become the only known treatment that appears to decrease the poor pregnancy outcome in PCOS women to date. The impact of using metformin as an adjunct to controlled ovarian stimulation and IVF also is promising and requires additional investigation particularly in women with of increased PAI-1 levels due to 4G/5G polymorphism.

Correlation between the increased PAI-1 levels and the suggestive findings of improved pregnancy outcome with metformin use supports the proposed pathogenic role of PAI-1 in early pregnancy complications. That forces extended metformin application in connection with increasing amount of data support for the safe use of metformin throughout pregnancy [147, 148], and because of the absence of reports for any drug's related teratogenicity effects [148], and also very low side effect incidences.

8. Other anticoagulant drugs instead LMWH

Fondaparinux is a synthetic pentasaccharide, a direct Factor Xa inhibitor. Fondaparinux forms a high affinity binding site for the anti-coagulant factor antithrombin III (ATIII). Binding to ATIII has been shown to increase the anti-coagulant activity of antithrombin III 1000 fold. In contrast to heparin, fondaparinux does not inhibit thrombin. Limited case-reports studies have shown effective treatment of inherited thrombophilia (Protein S deficiency) using Fondaparinux in case of heparin intolerance [149]. In situations where pregnant women cannot receive LMWH, fondaparinux may be a valuable alternative during pregnancy. Fetal safety is always an issue when considering maternal pharmacologic treatment. In a recently published report, a minor transplacental passage of fondaparinux was found in vivo [150] but until larger scale studies are available, the use of fondaparinux in pregnant women should be limited to those patients with either severe allergic reactions to heparin, or eventually to those with HIT.

Lepirudin and bivalirudin are anticoagulants, with parenteral action that functions as direct thrombin inhibitors. Direct Thrombin Inhibitors are recombinant derivats of hirudin. Lepirudin may be used as an anticoagulant when heparins (unfractionated or LMWH) are contraindicated because of heparin-induced thrombocytopenia. For pregnant women, ACCP [117] suggest limiting the use of fondaparinux and parenteral direct thrombin inhibitors to those with severe allergic reactions to heparin who cannot receive danaparoid.

Dabigatran, an oral anticoagulant from the class of the direct thrombin inhibitors does not require frequent blood tests for international normalized ratio (INR) monitoring while offering similar results in terms of efficacy like indirect anticoagulants. Clinical experience is lacking in populations for whom anticoagulants are routinely used, such as patients with pregnancy-associated thrombosis.

Rivaroxaban and apixaban are oral anticoagulants, the first available orally as active direct factor Xa inhibitors. Rivaroxaban is well absorbed from the gut and maximum inhibition of factor Xa occurs four hours after a dose. Rivaroxaban is a highly selective direct Factor Xa inhibitor with oral bioavailability and rapid onset of action. ACCP [117] recommends avoiding the use of oral direct thrombin (dabigatran) and anti-Xa (rivaroxaban, apixaban) inhibitors during pregnancy needing thromboprophylaxis.

9. Closing remarks

The maternal risk during pregnancy was increased with increments in the rates of recurrent pregnancy loss leading to placenta praevia, cervical incompetence, and consequently need for Caesarean section. All of these conditions are being increasingly recognized as having their origins in the first trimester. The abnormal implantation and trophoblast development have had the key role in these severe obstetrics complications. So endorsement of complicated due to inherited thrombophilic factor presence IVF achieved pregnancy in its very early stage of development could improve maternal as well as fetal outcome.

A couple of studies have shown a significant increase in the implantation and pregnancy rates after IVF procedures when use LMWH compared with those who did not. Although the process of implantation is not well understood, anticoagulant therapy is now being examined as a preventative measure for women undergoing IVF. Given the increased risk of adverse outcome associated with ART pregnancies, clinics commence to use LMWH, again based on biological plausibility rather than evidence of efficacy. Presence of thrombophilic factors such as FII 20210 G>A or polymorphisms 4G/5G in PAI-1 is desirable condition for LMWH prophylaxis even immediately after embryo transfer. Distinctly, presence of 4G allele in PAI-1 gene is suggestion to metformin complement also not only in PCO patients with insulin resistance but in all 4G allele carriers. In FVL carriers, the postpone of LMWH could be considered till positive pregnancy test, because of suspicious positive effect of the mutation on the implantation process. A ten-time increased dose of folic acid supplementation should be applicated even before the start of COH in MTHFR 677 TT genotype carriers to ensure not only better implantation chances but also improved follicular development during ovarian stimulation. Despite the found increased alphaV/beta3 integrin expression in the uterine endometrium in aspirin presence and separately raised acetylsalicylic acid resistance in beta3 polymorphism A1/A2 presence, the need for application and dose adjustment in the polymorphism apearance is still not clarified. An upcoming prospective randomized trial on LMWH and other supplement therapy would support scientific evidence for future clinical applications of medicines possibly related with after-IVF implantation outcome in inherited thrombophilia presence.

Author details

P. Ivanov[1], Sl. Tomov[2], Tsv. Tsvyatkovska[3], E. Konova[4,5] and R. Komsa-Penkova[6]

1 Clinical Institute for Reproductive Medicine, Department of Biochemistry, Medical University of Pleven, Pleven, Bulgaria

2 Deparment of Oncogynecology, Medical University of Pleven, Pleven, Bulgaria

3 Department of Biochemistry, Medical University of Pleven, Pleven, Bulgaria

4 Clinical Institute for Reproductive Medicine, Pleven, Pleven, Bulgaria

5 Center of Clinical Immunology, University Hospital of Pleven, Pleven, Bulgaria

6 Department of Biochemistry, Medical University of Pleven, Pleven, Bulgaria

References

[1] Nyboe Andersen A, Goossens V, Bhattacharya S, Ferraretti AP, Kupka MS, de Mouzon J, Nygren KG. Assisted reproductive technology and intrauterine inseminations in Europe, 2005: results generated from European registers by ESHRE: ESHRE. The European IVF Monitoring Programme (EIM), for the European Society of Human Reproduction and Embryology (ESHRE). Hum Reprod 2009;24:1267–1287.

[2] Society for Reproductive Technology: Clinic summary report. Available at: https://www.sartcorsonline.com/rptCSR_PublicMultYear. Accessed January 9, 2008.

[3] Qublan HS, Malkawi HY, Tahat YA, Areidah S, Nusair B, Khreisat BM, Al-Quraan G, Abu-Assaf A, Hadaddein MF, Abu-Jassar H. In-vitro fertilisation treatment: factors affecting its results and outcome. J Obstet Gynaecol 2005;25:689-693.

[4] Kovacs P, Matyas S, Boda K, Kaali S. The effect of endometrial thickness on IVF/ICSI outcome. Hum Reprod 2003 ;18:2337-2341.

[5] Stylianou C, Critchlow D, Brison DR, Roberts SA. Embryo morphology as a predictor of IVF success: An evaluation of the proposed UK ACE grading scheme for cleavage stage embryos. Hum Fertil (Camb). 2012;15:11-7.

[6] Kawato H, Tabata T, Minoura H, Murabayashi N, Ma N, Wang DF, Sagawa N: Factor XII gene expression in endometrial stromal cells during decidualisation. Reprod Fertil Dev 2009;21:840-847.

[7] Middeldorp S. Evidence-based approach to thrombophilia testing. J Thromb Thrombolysis 2011;31:275-278.

[8] Rosendaal FR. Venous thrombosis: a multicausal disease. Lancet 1999;353:1167–1173.

[9] Munne S, Lee A, Rosenwak Z, Grifo J, Cohen. Diagnosis of major chromosome aneuploidies in human preimplantation embryos. Hum Reprod 1993;8:2185–2191.

[10] Lipe B, Ornstein DL: Deficiencies of natural anticoagulants, protein C, protein S, and antithrombin. Circulation. 2011;124:365-368.

[11] Cacciapuoti F. Some considerations about the hypercoagulable states and their treatments.Blood Coagul Fibrinolysis 2011;22:155-159.

[12] Segers K, Dahlback B, Nicolaes GA. Coagulation factor V and thrombophilia: background and mechanisms. Thromb Haemost 2007;98:530-542.

[13] Rees DC, Cox M, Clegg JB. World distribution of factor V Leiden. Lancet 1995;346:1133-1134.

[14] Brenner B, Sarig G, Weiner Z et al. Thrombophilic polymorphisms are common in women with fetal loss without apparent cause. Thromb Haemost 1999; 82:6–9.

[15] Carp H, Salomon O, Seidman D, et al. Prevalence of genetic markers for thrombophilia in recurrent pregnancy loss. Hum Reprod 2002;17:1633–1637.

[16] Reznikoff-Etievan MF, Cayol V, Carbonne B. Factor V Leiden and G20210A prothrombin mutations are risk factors for very early recurrent miscarriage. BJOG 2001;108:1251–1254.

[17] Younis JS, Brenner B, Ohel G, et al. Activated protein C resistance and factor V Leiden mutation can be associated with fi rst- as well as secondtrimester recurrent pregnancy loss. Am J Reprod Immunol 2000;43:31–35.

[18] Rey E, Kahn SR, David M, Shrier I. Thrombophilic disorders and fetal loss: a meta-analysis. Lancet 2003;361:901–908.

[19] Robertson L, Wu O, Greer I. Thrombophilia and adverse pregnancy outcome. Curr Opin Obstet Gynecol 2004;16:453–458.

[20] Murphy RP, Donoghue C, Nallen RJ, D'Mello M, Regan C, Whitehead AS, Fitzgerald DJ. Prospective evaluation of the risk conferred by factor V Leiden and thermolabile methylenetetrahydrofolate reductase polymorphisms in pregnancy. Arterioscler Thromb Vasc Biol 2000;20:266–270.

[21] Dizon-Townson D, Miller C, Sibai B, Spong CY, Thom E, Wendel G, Jr, Wenstrom K, Samuels P, Cotroneo MA, Moawad A et al. The relationship of the factor V Leiden mutation and pregnancy outcomes for mother and fetus. Obstet Gynecol 2005;106:517–524.

[22] Goodman C, Jeyendran RS, Coulam CB. P53 tumor suppressor factor, plasminogen activator inhibitor, and vascular endothelial growth factor gene polymorphisms and recurrent implantation failure. Fertil Steril 2009;92:494-498.

[23] Coulam CB, Jeyendran RS, Fishel LA, Roussev R. Multiple thrombophilic gene mutations are risk factors for implantation failure. Reprod Biomed Online 2006;12:322-327.

[24] Qublan HS, Eid SS, Ababneh HA, Amarin ZO, Smadi AZ, Al-Khafaji FF, Khader YS. Acquired and inherited thrombophilia: implication in recurrent IVF and embryo transfer failure. Hum Reprod 2006;21:2694-2698.

[25] Enders AC, Schlafke S, Hendrickx AG. Differentiation of the embryonic disc, amnion, and yolk sac in the rhesus monkey. Am J Anat 1986;177:161-185.

[26] Lessey BA. Assessment of endometrial receptivity. Fertil Steril. 2011;96:522-529.

[27] Margadant C, Monsuur HN, Norman JC, Sonnenberg A. Mechanisms of integrin activation and trafficking. Curr Opin Cell Biol. 2011;23:607-614.

[28] Lessey BA. Embryo quality and endometrial receptivity: lessons learned from the ART experience. J Assist Reprod Genet. 1998;15:173–176.

[29] Lessey BA, Damjanovich L, Coutifaris C, Castelbaum A, Albelda SM, Buck CA: Integrin adhesion molecules in the human endometrium. Correlation with the normal and abnormal menstrual cycle. J Clin Invest 1992;90:188–195.

[30] Lessey BA. Endometrial integrins and the establishment of uterine receptivity. Hum. Reprod. 1998;13, 247–258.

[31] Sajid M, Vijayan KV, Souza S, Bray PF. PlA polymorphism of integrin β3 differentially modulates cellular migration on extracellular matrix proteins. Arterioscler Thromb Vasc Biol 2002;22:1984–1989.

[32] Liu J, Chakraborty C, Graham CH, Barbin YP, Dixon SJ & Lala PK. Noncatalytic domain of uPA stimulates human extravillous trophoblast migration by using phospholipase C, phosphatidylinositol 3-kinase and mitogen-activated protein kinase. Experimental Cell Research 2003;286:138–151.

[33] Staun-Ram E, Goldman S, Gabarin D, Shalev E. Expression and importance of matrix metalloproteinase 2 and 9 (MMP-2 and -9) in human trophoblast invasion. Reprod Biol Endocrinol 2004;2:59

[34] LaMarca HL, Ott CM, Höner Zu Bentrup K, Leblanc CL, Pierson DL, Nelson AB, Scandurro AB, Whitley GS, Nickerson CA, Morris CA. Three-dimensional growth of extravillous cytotrophoblasts promotes differentiation and invasion. Placenta 2005;26:709-712.

[35] Varanou A, Withington SL, Lakasing L, Williamson C, Burton GJ, Hemberger M. The importance of cysteine cathepsin proteases for placental development 2006;84:305-317.

[36] Blasi F, Carmeliet P. uPAR: a versatile signalling orchestrator. Nat Rev Mol Cell Biol 2002; 3:932–943.

[37] Ye S, Green FR, Scarabin PY, Nicaud V, Bara L, Dawson SJ, Humphries SE, Evans A, Luc G, Cambou JP, et al. The 4G/5G genetic polymorphism in the promoter of the plasminogen activator inhibitor-1 (PAI-1) gene is associated with differences in plasma PAI-1 activity but not with risk of myocardial infarction in the ECTIM study. Etude CasTemoins de I'nfarctus du Mycocarde. Thromb Haemost 1995;74:837-841.

[38] Eriksson P, Kallin B, van 't Hooft FM, Båvenholm P, Hamsten A. Allele-specific increase in basal transcription of the plasminogen-activator inhibitor 1 gene is associated with myocardial infarction. Proc Natl Acad Sci U S A 1995;92:1851-1855.

[39] Tsantes AE, Nikolopoulos GK, Bagos PG, Rapti E, Mantzios G, Kapsimali V, Travlou A. Association between the plasminogen activator inhibitor-1 4G/5G polymorphism and venous thrombosis. A meta-analysis. Thromb Haemost 2007;97:907-913.

[40] Cartwright JE, Fraser R, Leslie K, Wallace AE, James JL: Remodelling at the maternal-fetal interface: relevance to human pregnancy disorders. Reproduction 2010;140:803-813.

[41] Lockwood CJ, Krikun G, Rahman M, Caze R, Buchwalder L, Schatz F: The role of decidualization in regulating endometrial hemostasis during the menstrual cycle, gestation, and in pathological states. Semin Thromb Hemost 2007;33:111-117.

[42] Poort SR, Rosendaal FR, Reitsma PH, Bertina RM. A. Common genetic variation in the 3'-untranslated region of the prothrombin gene is associated with elevated plasma prothrombin levels and an increase in venous thrombosis. Blood. 1996;88:3698-3703.

[43] Razin A, Shemer R. DNA methylation in early development. Hum Mol Genet. 1995;4:1751-1755.

[44] Shi W, Haaf T. Aberrant methylation patterns at the two-cell stage as an indicator of early developmental failure. Mol Reprod Dev. 2002;63:329-334.

[45] Lucock M, Daskalakis I, Briggs D, Yates Z, Levene M. Altered folate metabolism and disposition in mothers affected by a spina bifida pregnancy: influence of 677c --> t methylenetetrahydrofolate reductase and 2756a --> g methionine synthase genotypes. Mol Genet Meta 2000;70:27-44.

[46] Duthie SJ, Narayanan S, Blum S, Pirie L, Brand GM. Folate deficiency in vitro induces uracil misincorporation and DNA hypomethylation and inhibits DNA excision repair in immortalized normal human colon epithelial cells. Nutr Cancer 2000;37:245-251.

[47] Castro R, Rivera I, Ravasco P, Camilo ME, Jakobs C, Blom HJ, de Almeida IT. 5,10-methylenetetrahydrofolate reductase (MTHFR) 677C-->T and 1298A-->C mutations are associated with DNA hypomethylation. J Med Gene. 2004;41:454-458.

[48] Robien K, Ulrich CM. 5,10-Methylenetetrahydrofolate reductase polymorphisms and leukemia risk: a HuGE minireview. Am J Epidemiol 2003;157:571-582.

[49] Nelen WL, Blom HJ, Thomas CM, Steegers EA, Boers GH, Eskes TK. Methylenetetrahydrofolate reductase polymorphism affects the change in homocysteine and folate concentrations resulting from low dose folic acid supplementation in women with unexplained recurrent miscarriages. J Nutr 1998;128:1336-1341.

[50] Isotalo PA, Wells GA, Donnelly JG: Neonatal and fetal methylenetetrahydrofolate reductase genetic polymorphisms: an examination of C677T and A1298C mutations. Am J Hum Genet 2000;67:986-990.

[51] Zetterberg H, Regland B, Palmér M, Ricksten A, Palmqvist L, Rymo L, Arvanitis DA, Spandidos DA, Blennow K. Increased frequency of combined methylenetetrahydrofolate reductase C677T and A1298C mutated alleles in spontaneously aborted embryos. Eur J Hum Genet. 2002;10:113-118.

[52] Kang SS, Zhou J, Wong PW, Kowalisyn J, Strokosch G. Intermediate homocysteinemia: a thermolabile variant of methylenetetrahydrofolate reductase. Am J Hum Genet 1988;43:414-421.

[53] Guenther BD, Sheppard CA, Tran P, Rozen R, Matthews RG, Ludwig ML. The structure and properties of methylenetetrahydrofolate reductase from Escherichia coli suggest how folate ameliorates human hyperhomocysteinemia. Nat Struct Biol 1999;6:359-365.

[54] Szymański W, Kazdepka-Ziemińska A. Effect of homocysteine concentration in follicular fluid on a degree of oocyte maturity. Ginekol Pol 2003;74:1392-1396.

[55] Dobson AT, Davis RM, Rosen MP, Shen S, Rinaudo PF, Chan J, Cedars MI. Methylenetetrahydrofolate reductase C677T and A1298C variants do not affect ongoing pregnancy rates following IVF. Hum Reprod. 2007;22:450-456.

[56] Heby O. DNA methylation and polyamines in embryonic development and cancer. Int J Dev Biol 1995;39:737–757.

[57] Nelen WLDM, Bulten J, Steegers EAP, Blom HJ, Hanselaar AGJ, Eskes TKAB. Maternal homocystine and chorionic vascularization in recurrent early pregnancy loss. Hum Reprod. 2000;15:953–960.

[58] Martinelli I, Taioli E, Ragni G, Levi-Setti P, Passamonti SM, Battaglioli T, Lodigiani C, Mannucci PM. Embryo implantation after assisted reproductive procedures and maternal thrombophilia. Haematologica 2003;88:789-793.

[59] Azem F, Many A, Ben Ami I, Yovel I, Amit A, Lessing JB, Kupferminc MJ. Increased rates of thrombophilia in women with repeated IVF failures. Hum Reprod 2004;19:368-370.

[60] Ivanov P, Komsa-Penkova R, Kovacheva K, Konova E, Todorova K, Simeonova M, Ivanov I, Stoĭkov S, Popov I, Tanchev S, Bozhinova S. Risk of thrombophilia in carriers of thrombophilic genetic factors in unsuccessful assisted reproduction. Akush Ginekol (Sofiia) 2007;46:3-8.

[61] Qin X, Li J, Cui Y, Liu Z, Zhao Z, Ge J, Guan D, Hu J, Wang Y, Zhang F, Xu X, Wang X, Xu X, Huo Y. MTHFR C677T and MTR A2756G polymorphisms and the homocysteine lowering efficacy of different doses of folic acid in hypertensive Chinese adults. Nutr J 2012 ;11:2.

[62] Crider KS, Quinlivan EP, Berry RJ, Hao L, Li Z, Maneval D, Yang TP, Rasmussen SA, Yang Q, Zhu JH, Hu DJ, Bailey LB. Genomic DNA methylation changes in response to folic acid supplementation in a population-based intervention study among women of reproductive age. PLoS One 2011;6: 28144.

[63] Rimm EB, Stampfer MJ. Folate and cardiovascular disease: one size does not fit all. Lancet. 2011;378:544-546.

[64] Lockwood CJ, Toti P, Arcuri F, Norwitz E, Funai EF, Huang ST, Buchwalder LF, Krikun G, Schatz F.Thrombin regulates soluble fms-like tyrosine kinase-1 (sFlt-1) expression in first trimester decidua: implications for preeclampsia. Am J Pathol 2007 ; 170:1398-1405.

[65] Rouselle D, Jarrel J, Belbeck L, Andryjowicz E, Hibbert P, McMahon A. Thrombin as an adjuvant to reanastomosis of the fallopian tubes reduces implantations in the rabbit. Can J Surg 1988;31:66-8.

[66] Ivanov PD, Komsa-Penkova RS, Konova EI, Kovacheva KS, Simeonova MN, Popov JD. Association of inherited thrombophilia with embryonic and postembryonic recurrent pregnancy loss. Blood Coagul Fibrinolysis 2009;20:134–140.

[67] Clark P, Brennand J, Conkie JA, McCall F, Greer IA and Walker ID. Activated Protein C Sensitivity, Protein C, Protein S and Coagulation in Normal Pregnancy. Thromb Haemost 1998;79:1166–1170.

[68] Grandone E, Colaizzo D, Lo Bue A, Checola MG, Cittadini E, Margaglione M. Inherited thrombophilia and in vitro fertilization implantation failure. Fertil Steril 2001;76:201-202.

[69] Simur A, Ozdemir S, Acar H, Colakoğlu MC, Görkemli H, Balci O, Nergis S. Repeated in vitro fertilization failure and its relation with thrombophilia. Gynecol Obstet Invest 2009;67:109-112.

[70] Göpel W, Ludwig M, Junge AK, Kohlmann T, Diedrich K, Möller J. Selection pressure for the factor-V-Leiden mutation and embryo implantation. Lancet 2001;358:1238-1239.

[71] Toth B, Vocke F, Rogenhofer N, Friese K, Thaler CJ, Lohse P. Paternal thrombophilic gene mutations are not associated with recurrent miscarriage. Am J Reprod Immunol 2008;60:325-332.

[72] Juul K, Tybjaerg-Hansen A, Nordestgaard BG. Factor V Leiden: relation to fertility? Lancet 2002;359:894.

[73] Lang IM, Moster KM, Schleef RR. Elevated expression of urokinase-like plasminogen activator and plasminogen activator inhibitor type 1 during the vascular remodeling associated with pulmonary thromboembolism. Arterioscler Thromb Vasc Biol 1998;18:808-815.

[74] Gris JC, Ripart-Neveu S, Maugard C, Tailland ML, Brun S, Courtieu C, Biron C, Hoffet M, Hédon B, Marès P. Respective evaluation of the prevalence of haemostasis abnormalities in unexplained primary early recurrent miscarriages. The Nimes Obstetricians and Haematologists (NOHA) Study. Thromb Haemost 1997;77:1096-1103.

[75] Dzhandzhgava ZhG, Bitsadze VO. IVF failures: maternal thrombophilia as a possible cause. Georgian Med News. 2005;124-125:23-26.

[76] Lambrinoudaki I, Armeni E, Kaparos GJ, Christodoulakos GE, Sergentanis TN, Alexandrou A, Creatsa M, Kouskouni E. The frequency of early, spontaneous miscarriage associated with the leu33pro polymorphism of Glycoprotein IIIa: a pilot study. Aust N Z J Obstet Gynaecol 2010;50:485-490.

[77] Ivanov PD, Komsa-Penkova RS, Konova EI, Tsvyatkovska TM, Kovacheva KS, Si-
      meonova MN, Tanchev SY. Polymorphism A1/A2 in the cell surface integrin subunit
      β3 and disturbance of implantation and placentation in women with recurrent preg-
      nancy loss. Fertil Steril 2010;94:2843-2845.

[78] Nardo LG, Bartoloni G, Di Mercurio S, Nardo F. Expression of alpha(v)beta3 and al-
      pha4beta1 integrins throughout the putative window of implantation in a cohort of
      healthy fertile women. Acta Obstet Gynecol Scand 2002;81:753-758.

[79] Kay C, Jeyendran RS, Coulam CB. P53 tumour suppressor polymorphism is associat-
      ed with recurrent implantation failure. Reprod Biomed Online. 2006;13:492–496.

[80] Goodman C, Jeyendran RS, Coulam CB. Vascular endothelial growth factor gene
      polymorphisms and recurrent implantation failure. Reprod Biomed Online
      2008;16:720–727.

[81] Zhao M, Chang C, Liu Z, Chen LM, Chen Q. Treatment with low-dose aspirin in-
      creased the level LIF and integrin β3 expression in mice during the implantation win-
      dow. Placenta 2010;31:1101-1105.

[82] Tranquilli AL, Saccucci F, Giannubilo SR, Cecati M, Nocchi L, Lorenzi S, Emanuelli
      M. Unexplained fetal loss: the fetal side of thrombophilia. Fertil Steril
      2010;94:378-380.

[83] Nelson SM, Greer IA. The potential role of heparin in assisted conception. Hum Re-
      prod Update 2008;14, 623–645.

[84] Fiedler K, Wurfel W. Effectivity of heparin in assisted reproduction. Eur J Med Res.
      2004;9;207–214.

[85] Genbacev OD, Prakobphol A, Foulk RA, Krtolica AR, Ilic D, Singer MS, Yang ZQ,
      Kiessling LL, Rosen SD, Fisher SJ. Trophoblast L-selectinmediated adhesion at the
      maternal–fetal interface. Science 2003;299:405–408.

[86] Stevenson JL, Choi SH, Varki A. Differential metastasis inhibition by clinically rele-
      vant levels of heparins—correlation with selectin inhibition, not antithrombotic activ-
      ity. Clin Cancer Res 2005;11:7003–7011.

[87] Cavallaro U, Christofori G. Cell adhesion and signalling by cadherins and Ig-CAMs
      in cancer. Nat Rev Cancer 2004;4:118–132.

[88] Jha RK, Titus S, Saxena D, Kumar PG, Laloraya M. Profiling of E-cadherin, [beta]-cat-
      enin and Ca2+in embryo–uterine interactions at implantation. FEBS Lett
      2006;580:5653–5660.

[89] Erden O, Imir A, Guvenal T, Muslehiddinoglu A, Arici S, Cetin M, Cetin A. Investi-
      gation of the effects of heparin and low molecular weight heparin on E-cadherin and
      laminin expression in rat pregnancy by immunohistochemistry. Hum Reprod
      2006;21:3014–3018.

[90] Iwamoto R, Mekada E. Heparin-binding EGF-like growth factor: a juxtacrine growth factor. Cytokine Growth Factor Rev 2000;11:335–344.

[91] Martin KL, Barlow DH, Sargent IL. Heparin-binding epidermal growth factor significantly improves human blastocyst development and hatching in serum-free medium. Hum Reprod 1998;13:1645–1652.

[92] Leach RE, Kilburn B, Wang J, Liu Z, Romero R, Armant DR. Heparin-binding EGF-like growth factor regulates human extravillous cytotrophoblast development during conversion to the invasive phenotype. Dev Biol 2004;266:223–237.

[93] Fowden AL. The insulin-like growth factors and feto–placental growth. Placenta 2003;24:803–812.

[94] Bach LA, Headey SJ, Norton RS. IGF-binding proteins—the pieces are falling into place. Trends Endocrinol Metab 2005;16:228–234.

[95] MollerAV, Jorgensen SP,ChenJW, Larnkjaer A, Ledet T, Flyvbjerg A, Frystyk J. Glycosaminoglycans increase levels of free and bioactive IGF-I in vitro. Eur J Endocrinol 2006;155:297–305.

[96] Lash GE, Otun HA, Innes BA, Bulmer JN, Searle RF, Robson SC. Inhibition of trophoblast cell invasion by TGFB1, 2, and 3 is associated with a decrease in active proteases. Biol Reprod 2005;73:374–381.

[97] Pecly IMD,Goncalves RG, Rangel EP, Takiya CM, Taboada FS, Martinusso CA, Pavao MSG, Leite M, Jr. Effects of low molecular weight heparin in obstructed kidneys: decrease of collagen, fibronectin and TGF-gbetaf, and increase of chondroitin/dermatan sulfate proteoglycans and macrophage infiltration. Nephrol Dial Transplant 2006;21:1212–1222.

[98] Lavranos TC, Rathjen PD, Seamark RF. Trophic effects of myeloid leukaemia inhibitory factor (LIF) on mouse embryos. J Reprod Fertil 1995;105:331–338.

[99] Simon C, Gimeno MJ, Mercader A, O'Connor JE, Remohi J, Polan ML, Pellicer A. Embryonic regulation of integrins beta 3, alpha 4, and alpha 1 in human endometrial epithelial cells in vitro. J Clin Endocrinol Metab 1997;82:2607–2616.

[100] Call DR, Remick DG. Low molecular weight heparin is associated with greater cytokine production in a stimulated whole blood model. Shock 1998;10:192–197.

[101] Dimitriadis E, Stoikos C, Baca M, Fairlie WD, McCoubrie JE, Salamonsen LA. Relaxin and prostaglandin E2 regulate interleukin 11 during human endometrial stromal cell decidualization. J Clin Endocrinol Metab 2005;90:3458–3465.

[102] Dimitriadis E, Stoikos C, Stafford-Bell M, Clark I, Paiva P, Kovacs G, Salamonsen LA. Interleukin-11, IL-11 receptor[alpha] and leukemia inhibitory factor are dysregulated in endometrium of infertile women with endometriosis during the implantation window. J Reprod Immunol 2006;69:53–64.

[103] Dimitriadis E, White CA, Jones RL, Salamonsen LA. Cytokines, chemokines and growth factors in endometrium related to implantation. Hum Reprod Update 2005;11:613–630.

[104] Gutierrez G, Sarto A, Berod L, Canellada A, Gentile T, Pasqualini S, Margni RA. Regulation of interleukin-6 fetoplacental levels could be involved in the protective effect of low-molecular weight heparin treatment on murine spontaneous abortion. Am J Reprod Immunol 2004;51:160–165.

[105] Robertson SA. GM-CSF regulation of embryo development and pregnancy. Cytokine Growth Factor Rev 2007;18:287–298.

[106] Liang A, Du Y, Wang K, Lin B. Quantitative investigation of the interaction between granulocyte-macrophage colony-stimulating factor and heparin by capillary zone electrophoresis. J Sep Sci 2006;29:1637–1641.

[107] Niu R, Okamoto T, Iwase K, Nomura S, Mizutani S. Quantitative analysis of matrix metalloproteinases-2 and -9, and their tissue inhibitors-1 and -2 in human placenta throughout gestation. Life Sci 2000;66:1127–1137.

[108] Dubois B, Arnold B, Opdenakker G. Gelatinase B deficiency impairs reproduction. J Clin Invest 2000;106:627–628.

[109] Xu P, Wang YL, Zhu SJ, Luo SY, Piao YS, Zhuang LZ. Expression of matrix metalloproteinase-2, -9, and -14, tissue inhibitors of metalloproteinase-1, and matrix proteins in human placenta during the first trimester. Biol Reprod 2000;62:988–994.

[110] Di Simone N, Di Nicuolo F, Sanguinetti M, Ferrazzani S, D'Alessio MC, Castellani R, Bompiani A, Caruso A. Low-molecular weight heparin induces in vitro trophoblast invasiveness: role of matrix metalloproteinases and tissue inhibitors. Placenta 2007;28:298–304.

[111] Bellver J, Soares SR, Alvarez C, Muñoz E, Ramírez A, Rubio C, Serra V, Remohí J, Pellicer A: The role of thrombophilia and thyroid autoimmunity in unexplained infertility, implantation failure and recurrent spontaneous abortion. Hum Reprod 2008;23:278-284.

[112] Coulam CB: Implantation failure and immunotherapy. Hum Reprod 1995;10:1338–1340.

[113] Qublan H, Amarin Z, Dabbas M et al. Low-molecular-weight heparin in the treatment of recurrent IVF-ET failure and thrombophilia: a prospective randomized placebo-controlled trial. Hum Fertil (Camb.) 2008;11:246–253.

[114] Ricci G, Giolo E, Simeone R. Heparin's 'potential to improve pregnancy rates and outcomes' is not evidence-based. Hum Reprod Update 2010;16:225-7.

[115] Urman B, Ata B, Yakin K et al. Luteal phase empirical low molecular weight heparin administration in patients with failed ICSI embryo transfer cycles: a randomized open-labeled pilot trial. Hum. Reprod 2009;24:1640–1647.

[116] Lodigiani C, Di Micco P, Ferrazzi P, Librè L, Arfuso V, Polatti F, Benigna M, Rossini R, Morenghi E, Rota L, Brenner B, Setti PE. Low-molecular-weight heparin in women with repeated implantation failure. Womens Health (Lond Engl) 2011;7:425-31.

[117] Bates SM, Greer IA, Middeldorp S, Veenstra DL, Prabulos AM, Vandvik PO; American College of Chest Physicians. VTE, thrombophilia, antithrombotic therapy, and pregnancy: Antithrombotic Therapy and Prevention of Thrombosis, 9th ed: American College of Chest Physicians Evidence-Based Clinical Practice Guidelines. Chest. 2012;141(2 Suppl):e691S-736S.

[118] Rey E, David M. The use of LMWH in pregnancies at risk: new evidence or perception? J Thromb Haemost 2005;3:782–783.

[119] Hunt BJ, Doughty H, Majumdar G et al. Thromboprophylaxis with low molecular weight heparin (Fragmin) in high risk pregnancies. Thromb Haemost 1997;77:39–43.

[120] Kaandorp SP, Goddijn M, van der Post JA, Hutten BA, Verhoeve HR, Hamulyak K, Mol BW, Folkeringa N, Nahuis M, Papatsonis DN, BuË ller HR, van der Veen F, Middeldorp S. Aspirin plus heparin or aspirin alone in women with recurrent miscarriage. N Engl JMed 2010;362:1586–96.

[121] Casele HL, Laifer SA, Woelkers DA, Venkataramanan R. Changes in the pharmacokinetics of the low-molecular-weight heparin enoxaparin sodium during pregnancy. Am J Obstet Gynecol 1999;181:1113–1117.

[122] Ginsberg JS, Greer I, Hirsh J. Use of antithrombotic agents during pregnancy. Chest 2001;119:122S–131S.

[123] Brenner B, Bar J, Ellis M, Yarom I, Yohai D, Samueloff A; Live-Enox Investigators. Effects of enoxaparin on late pregnancy complications and neonatal outcome in women with recurrent pregnancy loss and thrombophilia: results from the Live-Enox study. Fertil Steril. 2005 Sep;84(3):770-3.

[124] Rowan JA, McLintock C, Taylor RS, North RA.Prophylactic and therapeutic enoxaparin during pregnancy: indications, outcomes and monitoring. Aust N Z J Obstet Gynaecol 2003;43:123-8.

[125] Li N, Hu H, Lindqvist M, Wikstrom-Jonsson E, Goodall AH, Hjemdahl P. Platelet-leukocyte cross talk in whole blood. Arterioscler Thromb Vasc Biol 2000;20:2702-2708.

[126] Lukanov TH, Veleva GL, Konova EI, Ivanov PD, Kovacheva KS, Stoykov DJ. Levels of platelet-leukocyte aggregates in women with both thrombophilia and recurrent pregnancy loss. Clin Appl Thromb Hemost 2011;17:181-7.

[127] Goswamy RK, Williams G, Steptoe PC. Decreased uterine perfusion—a cause of infertility. Hum Reprod 1988;3:955–959.

[128] Steer CV, Campbell S, Tan SL, Crayford T, Mills C, Mason BA, Collins WP. The use of transvaginal color flow imaging after in vitro fertilization to identify optimum uterine conditions before embryo transfer. Fertil Steril 1992;57:372–376.

[129] Arias F. Pharmacology of oxytocin and prostaglandins. Clin Obstet Gynecol 2000;43:455–468.

[130] Empson M, Lassere M, Craig J, Scott J. Prevention of recurrent miscarriage for women with antiphospholipid antibody or lupus anticoagulant. Cochrane Database Syst Rev 2005;18:CD002859.

[131] Lok IH, Yip SK, Cheung LP, Yin Leung PH, Haines CJ: Adjuvant low-dose aspirin therapy in poor responders undergoing in vitro fertilization: a prospective, randomized, double-blind, placebo-controlledtrial. Fertil Steril 2004;81:556-561.

[132] Lambers MJ, Mijatovic V, Hompes PG: Low dose aspirin and IVF: 'is it time for a meta-analysis'? Continued: the consequences of the choices made. Hum Reprod Update 2009;15:262-263.

[133] Weckstein LN, Jacobson A, Galen D, Hampton K, Hammel J: Low-dose aspirin for oocyte donation recipients with a thin endometrium: prospective, randomized study. Fertil Steril 1997;68:927-930.

[134] Waldenstrom U, Hellberg D, Nilsson S. Low-dose aspirin in a short regimen as standard treatment in in vitro fertilization: a randomized, prospective study. Fertil Steril 2004;81:1560–1564.

[135] Ruopp MD, Collins TC, Whitcomb BW, Schisterman EF: Evidence of absence or absence of evidence? A reanalysis of the effects of low-dose aspirin in in vitro fertilization. Fertil Steril 2008;90:71-76.

[136] Arias F, Romero R, Joist H, Kraus FT: Thrombophilia: a mechanism of disease in women with adverse pregnancy outcome and thrombotic lesions of the placenta. J Matern Fetal Med 1998;7:277-86.

[137] Szczeklik A, Undas A, Sanak M, Frolow M, Wegrzyn W: Relationship between bleeding time, aspirin and the PlA1/A2 polymorphism of platelet glycoprotein IIIa. Br J Haematol 2000;110:965-967.

[138] Pamukcu B, Oflaz H, Nisanci Y: The role of platelet glycoprotein IIIa polymorphism in the high prevalence of in vitro aspirin resistance in patients with intracoronary stent restenosis. Am Heart J 2005;149:675-680.

[139] Kosar A, Kasapoglu B, Kalyoncu S, Turan H, Balcik OS, Gümüs EI.Treatment of adverse perinatal outcome in inherited thrombophilias: a clinical study. Blood Coagul Fibrinolysis 2011;22:14-8.

[140] Siristatidis CS, Dodd SR, Drakeley AJ. Aspirin is not recommended for women undergoing IVF. Hum Reprod Update 2012;18:233.

[141] Nestler JE, Jakubowicz DJ, Evans WS, Pasquali R. Effects of metformin on spontaneous and clomiphine-induced ovulation in the polycystic ovary syndrome. N Engl J Med 1998;338:1876–1880.

[142] Ikeda T, Iwata K, Murakami H. Inhibitory effect of metformin on intestinal glucose absorption in the perfused rat intestine. Biochem Pharmacol 2000;59:887–890.

[143] Moghetti P, Castello R, Negri C, Tosi F, Perrone F, Caputo M, Zanolin E, Muggeo M. Metformin effects on clinical features, endocrine and metabolic profiles and insulin sensitivity in polycystric ovary syndrome: a radomized, double blind, placebo-controlled 6-month trial, followed by open, long-term clinical evaluation. J Clin Endocrinol Metab 2000;85:139–146.

[144] Attia GR, Rainey WE, Carr BR. Metformin directly inhibits androgen production in human thecal cells. Fertil. Steril 2001;76:517–524.

[145] He G, Pedersen SB, Bruun JM, Lihn AS, Richelsen B. Metformin, but not thiazolidinediones, inhibits plasminogen activator inhibitor-1 production in human adipose tissue in vitro. Horm Metab Res 2003;35:18-23.

[146] Glueck CJ, Sieve L, Zhu B, Wang P. Plasminogen activator inhibitor activity, 4G5G polymorphism of the plasminogen activator inhibitor 1 gene, and first-trimester miscarriage in women with polycystic ovary syndrome.Metabolism 2006;55:345-52.

[147] Glueck CJ,Wang P, Kobayashi S, Phillips H, Sieve-Smith L. Metformin therapy throughout pregnancy reduces the development of gestational diabetes in women with polycystic ovary syndrome. Fertil. Steril 2002;77: 520–525.

[148] Glueck CJ, Phillips H, Cameron D, Sieve-Smith L, Wang P. Continuing metformin throughout pregnancy in women with polycystic ovary syndrome appears to safely reduce first-trimester spontaneous abortion: a pilot study. Fertil. Steril 2001;75: 46–52.

[149] Mazzolai L, Hohlfeld P, Spertini F, Hayoz D, Schapira M, Duchosal MA. Fondaparinux is a safe alternative in case of heparin intolerance during pregnancy. Blood 2006;108:1569-70.

[150] Dempfle CE. Minor transplacental passage of fondaparinux in vivo. N Engl J Med 2004;350:1914-1915.

Chapter 7

Antiphospholipid Antibodies Syndrome and Reproductive Failures: New Therapeutic Trends Beyond Aspirin and Heparin

Chiara Tersigni, Silvia D'Ippolito and
Nicoletta Di Simone

Additional information is available at the end of the chapter

1. Introduction

The most investigated thrombophilia related to obstetrical complications is the antiphospholipid antibodies syndrome (APS), also known as Hughes' syndrome. APS is characterized by recurrent thrombosis (arterial or venous, or both) and/or morbidity during pregnancy (losses during early and late pregnancy and pre-eclampsia) associated with moderate to high plasma levels of antiphospholipid (aPL) antibodies (anticardiolipin antibodies, antibodies to β2 glycoprotein I [β2GPI] or lupus anticoagulants) [1-2].

According to the last International consensus statement for APS diagnostic criteria, in order to make diagnosis of the syndrome, the combination of at least one clinical and one laboratory criterion is required [2] (Table 1).

Since aPL antibodies have thrombogenic properties, intraplacental thrombosis with maternal–fetal blood exchange impairment was traditionally suggested to be the main pathogenic mechanism responsible of fetal loss in patients with APS, providing the rationale for the use of aspirin or heparin to prevent adverse pregnancy outcomes in APS [3-5].

Although the management of aPL antibodies-positive pregnant patients is controversial due to the limited well-designed controlled trials, the current recommendation is to use low-dose aspirin and prophylactic or therapeutic doses of heparin for patients fulfilling the updated Sapporo APS classification criteria [2] and no treatment for asymptomatic (no history of pregnancy complications and/or thrombosis) persistently aPL antibodies-positive patients [6].

Clinical criteria	Laboratory criteria
Vascular thrombosis • One or more clinical episodes of arterial, venous, or small vessel thrombosis, in any tissue or organ. • Thrombosis should be supported by objective validated criteria—ie, unequivocal findings of appropriate imaging studies or histopathology. For histopathological support, thrombosis should be present without substantial evidence of inflammation in the vessel wall. Pregnancy morbidity, defined by one of the following criteria: • One or more unexplained deaths of a morphologically healthy foetus at or beyond the 10th week of gestation, with healthy foetal morphology documented by ultrasound or by direct examination of the fetus. • One or more premature births of a morphologically healthy newborn baby before the 34th week of gestation because of: eclampsia or severe preeclampsia defined according to standard definitions or recognized features of placental failure. • Three or more unexplained consecutive spontaneous abortions before the 10th week of gestation, with maternal anatomical or hormonal abnormalities and paternal and maternal chromosomal causes excluded. In studies of populations of patients who have more than one type of pregnancy morbidity, investigators are strongly encouraged to stratify groups of patients according to one of the three criteria.	• Lupus anticoagulant present in plasma, on two or more occasions at least 12 weeks apart, detected according to the guidelines of the International Society on Thrombosis and Hemostasis (Scientific Subcommittee on lupus anticoagulant/ phospholipid-dependent antibodies). • Anticardiolipin antibody of IgG or IgM isotype, or both, in serum or plasma, present in medium or high titres (ie, "/>40 GPL or MPL, or greater than the 99th percentile) on two or more occasions, at least 12 weeks apart, measured by a standardized ELISA. • Anti-β2-gycoprotein 1 antibody of IgG or IgM isotype, or both, in serum or plasma (in titres greater than the 99th percentile), present on two or more occasions, at least 12 weeks apart, measured by a standardized ELISA, according to recommended procedures.

Table 1. Revised diagnostic criteria of APS [2].

In the last years, progress has been made in characterizing the molecular basis of aPL anti-bodies pathogenicity, which includes direct effects on platelets, endothelial cells and mono-cytes as well as activation of complement. Furthermore, it has been widely shown that pregnancy loss cannot be attributed exclusively to placental thrombosis and that other pathogenic mechanisms like functional trophoblast impairment, angiogenesis inhibition or complement-mediated placental injury may occur (see more below). Based on these findings, novel therapeutic targets are currently being explored for APS in order to address the unmet needs of better, safer and ideally targeted therapy.

This chapter points to resume the known mechanisms of aPL antibodies-mediated pregnancy impairment, the proven therapies and the new therapeutic perspectives to ameliorate obstetric outcomes of pregnant women with APS.

2. Adverse pregnancy outcomes associated to APS

Beyond thromboses, obstetric complications are the other main features of APS. Such associ-ation is supported by several epidemiological studies and experimental models showing that passive transfer of aPL IgG induces fetal losses and growth retardation in pregnant naive mice, giving the proof that aPL antibodies are involved in determining the clinical manifestations of the syndrome [7-9]. The most common adverse pregnancy outcome associated to APS is recurrent miscarriage, defined as the occurrence of three or more unexplained consecutive miscarriages before the 10th week of gestation. Other obstetric features of APS are unexplained fetal deaths, occurring at or beyond the 10th week of gestation, and premature births of a morphologically healthy newborn baby before the 34th week of gestation because of eclampsia or severe preeclampsia [10].

Recurrent miscarriage occurs in about 1% of the general population attempting to have children [11] and about 10–15% of women with recurrent miscarriage are diagnosed with APS [12,13]. Fetal death in the second or third trimesters of pregnancy occurs in up to 5% of unselected pregnancies [14] but it is less likely as pregnancy advances [15]. Although fetal death occurs significantly most often in APS [16], the overall contribution of this syndrome to its pathogenesis is unknown, because of the effect of other possible contributing factors such as underlying hypertension or pre-existing comorbidities, like systemic lupus erythematosus (SLE) or renal diseases. Furthermore, it has been observed that pregnant women with diagnosis of APS are at increased risk for developing preeclampsia or placental insufficiency.

Even if it is still unknown the precise relationship between aPL antibodies and the occurrence of obstetric complications, aPL antibodies seem to be detectable in 11–29% of women with preeclampsia, compared with 7% or less in controls and in 25% of women delivering growth restricted fetuses [17]. Furthermore, results from prospective cohort studies indicate that among pregnant women with high concentrations of aPL antibodies, 10–50% develop preeclampsia, and more than 10% of these women deliver infants who are small for gestational age [17].

A significant correlation between aPL positivity and increased risk of fetal loss has also been established. In particular, the strongest association has been observed with ACA positivity, followed by annexin V, lupus anticoagulant and anti-β2GPI. In addition, lupus anticoagulant seems to be significantly associated with early pregnancy loss compared to late pregnancy loss [18]

3. Pathogenetic mechanisms mediated by aPL antibodies and related therapeutic approaches

3.1. Vascular and placental thrombosis

The molecular mechanisms underlying thrombosis and fetal death in APS have long been investigated. The main target antigens reported in patients with APS include β2GPI/cardiolipin, prothrombin and annexin V [19]. Other putative antigens are thrombin, protein C, protein S, thrombomodulin, tissue plasminogen activator, kininogens (high or low molecular), prekallikrein, factor VII/VIIa, factor XI, factor XII, complement component C4, heparan sulfate proteoglycan, heparin, oxidised low-density lipoproteins [19,20]. The main autoantigens are attracted to negatively charged phospholipids exposed on the outer side of cell membranes in great amounts only under special circumstances such as damage or apoptosis (e.g. endothelial cell) or after activation (e.g. platelets) [19].

Endothelial cells, activated by aPL antibodies with anti-β2GPI activity, express adhesion molecules such as intercellular cell adhesion molecule-1, vascular cell adhesion molecule-1, E-selectin, and both endothelial cells and monocytes upregulate the production of tissue factor (TF) [21]. All at once, activated platelets increase expression of glycoprotein IIb-IIIa and synthesis of thromboxane A2, determining a procoagulant state [21-25].

Additional mechanisms promoting clot formation could be represented by interaction of aPL antibodies with proteins implicated in clotting regulation, such as annexin A5, prothrombin, factor X, protein C and plasmin [20,21,26].

Recent results from studies in mice highlight the role of inflammation in the pathogenesis of APS, showing a central role for complement activation in determining thrombosis and fetal loss induced by aPL antibodies [27,28]. Because many individuals with high aPL antibodies titers remain asymptomatic, a "second hit" hypothesis has been proposed. It is likely that in the aPL antibodies-induced vascular procoagulant state, activation of the complement cascade might close the loop and provoke thrombosis, often in the presence of a second hit, like tobacco, inflammation, or oestrogens [26,29,30].

Starting from the observation of the intravascular aPL antibodies-mediate clot formation, initially, intraplacental thrombosis was considered the main pathogenic mechanism mediating fetal loss in APS. This hypothesis of placental damage was supported by the finding of thrombosis and infarction in placentas from women with APS and by the demonstration of aPL antibodies capability to induce a procoagulant state in vitro through several mechanisms, including their ability (specifically, anti-β2GPI antibodies) to disrupt the anticoagulant annexin A5 shield on trophoblast and endothelial cell monolayers [20,31,32]. Supporting the in vitro findings, a significantly lower distribution of annexin A5 covering the intervillous surfaces was found in the placentas of aPL antibodies-positive women in comparison with normal controls [33]. These observations supported the introduction of heparin in the prevention of fetal loss in APS, preferred to oral anticoagulant therapies for its safer profile for the fetus. Indeed, it was demonstrated that heparin, at concentrations that are reached therapeutically in vivo, greatly enhanced the plasmin-mediated cleavage of β2-GPI. Considering that the cleaved forms of β2-GPI cannot bind to PL and may be cleared more rapidly from the circulation than native β2-GPI [34], interaction with heparin should greatly reduce the prothrombotic effects of anti-β2-GPI antibodies. Yet, some clinical trials confirmed heparin therapy effectiveness in improving pregnancy outcomes in APS patients [35].

Nevertheless, since recurrence of thrombotic events occurs despite the therapy and thrombosis cannot account for all of the histopathologic findings in placentae from women with APS, other mechanisms of reproductive impairment were supposed to be involved [36,37].

3.2. Defective placentation

3.2.1. Trophoblast invasiveness impairment

New aPL antibodies-mediated pathogenic mechanisms have been proposed during the last fifteen years: anti-β2GPI antibodies seem to bind directly the maternal decidua and the invading trophoblast, determining defective placentation.

On the fetal side, β2GPI has been shown to be expressed on trophoblast cell membranes, explaining the placental tropism of anti-β2GPI antibodies. Being a cationic plasma protein, β2GPI has been suggested to bind to exposed phosphatidylserine on the external cell membranes of trophoblasts undergoing syncitium formation [38].

β2GPI-dependent antibodies can adhere to human trophoblast cells in vitro [39], consistently with the hypothesis that the visibility of anionic PLs on the external cell surface during intertrophoblastic fusion might offer a useful substrate for the cation PL-binding site [40,41]. The binding to anionic structures induces the expression of new cryptic epitopes and/or increases the antigenic density, two events that are apparently pivotal for the antibody binding [42]. In vitro studies with both murine and human monoclonal antibodies, as well as with polyclonal IgG antibodies from APS patients, have clearly demonstrated a binding to trophoblast monolayers [39,43]. Interestingly, antibodies obtained from patients with APS, once bound, can affect the trophoblast functions in vitro, inducing cell injury and apoptosis, inhibition of proliferation and formation of syncitia, decreased production of human chorionic gonadotrophin, defective secretion of growth factors and impaired invasiveness [39]. β2GPI-dependent aPL antibodies seem, therefore, to represent the main pathogenic autoantibodies in obstetrical APS.

The most important mechanism by which heparin acts protecting placenta in APS seems to be its ability to prevent the binding of aPL antibodies to trophoblast cells. Indeed, using an expression/site-directed mutagenesis approach, Guerin demonstrated that the primary heparin-binding site of β2-GPI is the positively charged site located within the fifth domain of the protein, which also binds to PL [44]. Furthermore, we demonstrated that heparin reduces the aPL antibody binding to trophoblast cells in vitro and that it is able to restore placental invasiveness and differentiation [45,46].

Recent findings have underlined a further mechanism by which aPL antibodies binding to human trophoblast could affect its functions: the aPL antibodies-mediated reduction of placental Heparin-Binding Epidermal Growth Factor–like growth factor (HB-EGF) expression. HB-EGF is a member of the EGF family [47,48]. It has been shown to induce an invasive trophoblast phenotype in human and mouse blastocysts [49,50] and to initiate the molecular and cellular changes characteristic of decidualization in mice [51]. HB-EGF is expressed in the human placenta during the first trimester, primarily within the villous trophoblast, but also in the extravillous cytotrophoblast, predominantly at the sites of cytotrophoblast extravillous invasion [52]. Women with preeclampsia and infants small for gestational age display decreased placental expression of HB-EGF [53], strongly suggesting an association between HB-EGF down-regulation, poor trophoblast invasion, and failed physiologic transformation of the spiral arteries occurring in these disorders.

Interestingly, also in placental tissues obtained from women with APS, we found reduced expression of HB-EGF [54]. Furthermore, we showed that polyclonal and monoclonal aPL antibodies bind trophoblast monolayers in vitro significantly reducing the synthesis and the secretion of HB-EGF [55]. The ability of exogenous recombinant HB-EGF to reduce the aPL antibodies mediated effects on trophoblast cells supports the hypothesis of a key pathogenic role of this molecule in mediating APS-related adverse pregnancy outcomes.

We also observed that the addition of heparin inhibited aPL antibodies binding and restored HB-EGF expression in a dose-dependent manner [54]. These findings suggest that the reduction of aPL antibodies-mediated HB-EGF represents an additional mechanism that is responsible for the defective placentation associated with APS and provide one more proof that heparin works in protecting pregnancy from aPL antibodies-induced damage by inhibiting antibody binding to trophoblast cells.

3.2.2. Endometrial angiogenesis inhibition

On the maternal side, endometrial endothelial angiogenesis inhibition has been suggested to be a further aPL antibodies-mediated mechanism of placental damage. Indeed, aPL antibodies have been observed to selectively bind in vitro to endothelial cells isolated from human endometrium (HEEC) and to inhibit endothelial cell differentiation into capillary-like tubular structures, by reducing matrix metalloproteinase-2 (MMP-2) activity and vascular endothelial growth factor (VEGF) secretion, via a suppression of intracellular NFKB DNA binding activity [55]. Such an aPL antibodies-mediated inhibition of angiogenesis has also been confirmed in vivo in a murine model, showing a reduced angiogenesis in subcutaneous implanted angioreactors in aPL antibodies-inoculated mice [55]. Since it is well known that endometrial angiogenesis and decidualization are fundamental prerequisites for successful implantation and placental development, aPL antibodies-inhibition of this central process provides an important additional mechanism able to explain the association between APS and pregnancy complications associated to placental failure, like miscarriage, fetal growth restriction and preeclampsia.

Recently, we investigated whether two low molecular weight heparins (LMWHs), tinzaparin and enoxaparin, have an effect on the aPL antibodies-inhibited endometrial angiogenesis. We demonstrated that the addition of the two LMWHs prevents aPL antibodies-mediated inhibition of HEEC angiogenesis, both in vitro and in vivo in a murine model, and that LMWHs are able to restore Nuclear Factor-κB (NF-κB) and/or STAT-3 activity, VEGF secretion and MMP-2 activity inhibited by aPL antibodies [56]. A noteworthy aspect of our results was that tinzaparin improved aPL-inhibited in vitro angiogenesis and STAT-3 activity more effectively than enoxaparin but it is difficult to explain this difference between the two LMWHs and caution is necessary in extrapolating the obtained results.

In conclusion, this study provides the demonstration of a beneficial effect of LMWHs on the aPL antibodies-inhibited HEEC angiogenesis offering a new mechanism whereby treatment with heparin protects early pregnancy in APS.

Beyond heparin administration, recently, a new therapeutic perspective has been investigated to provide a safer profile therapy to prevent aPL antibodies-mediated angiogenesis inhibition. During the last decade, several groups attempted to neutralize the pathogenic effect of aPL antibodies by using synthetic peptides reproducing the β2GPI epitopes recognized by these antibodies [57,58].

An alternative approach by other groups employed synthetic portions of the whole molecule able to compete with β2GPI in its binding to the natural cell targets, ultimately inhibiting its expression and the recognition by specific autoantibodies [59,60]. It has been shown that a twenty amino acid synthetic peptide of viral origin spanning Thr101-Thr120 of ULB0-HCMVA from human Cytomegalovirus (TIFI) shares similarity with a 15 amino acid sequence rich in lysines in the Vth domain of β2GPI located in the PL-binding site [61]. TIFI inhibits the binding of FITC-conjugated β2GPI to human endothelial cells and murine monocytes in vitro. It has been demonstrated that this peptide is not recognized by aPL antibodies but it is able to reverse the aPL antibodies-mediated thrombosis in mice [59]. Furthermore, TIFI was recently shown to inhibit also the binding of monoclonal human β2GPI-dependent aPL antibodies to human trophoblast in vitro, and, more importantly, it has been observed that repeated injections of TIFI protected pregnant naïve mice from fetal loss and growth retardation induced by passive infusion of human aPL IgG [62-64]. Since β2GPI was shown to bind endothelial cells and trophoblasts through the PL-binding site, it has been suggested that TIFI might compete with β2GPI in the binding to cell membranes so reducing the amount of the target antigen available for aPL antibodies and ultimately might reverse the autoantibody-mediated pro-thrombotic or fetal loss effects [59,61-65] (Figure 1).

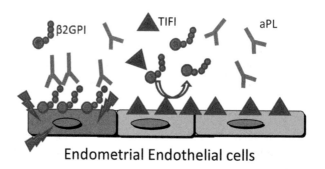

Figure 1. TIFI competes with β2GPI in the binding to HEEC membranes reducing the amount of the target antigen available for aPL antibodies and ultimately reverses the autoantibody-mediated fetal loss [66].

Based on these recent discoveries, we examined the ability of TIFI to interfere with aPL antibodies-mediated inhibition of human endometrial angiogenesis and we observed that the peptide is able to revert the anti-angiogenic effects mediated by a β2GPI-dependent aPL monoclonal IgG on HEEC both in vitro and in vivo [66]. We showed for the first time that TIFI is able to prevent the effects of β2GPI-dependent aPL antibodies on human endometrial endothelial cell (HEEC) functions. In fact, the addition of TIFI to HEEC cultures restores VEGF expression and MMP-2 gelatinolytic capacity affected by β2GPI-dependent monoclonal aPL antibodies [66]. This finding is also confirmed by parallel experiments performed in a murine model of in vivo angiogenesis [66].

3.3. Inflammation

A physiological pregnancy development requires a fine regulation of the maternal immune response during embryo implantation. Acute inflammatory events are recognized causes of adverse pregnancy outcomes, and proinflammatory mediators, such as complement, tumor necrosis factor (TNF), and CC chemokines, have been shown to play a role in animal models of aPL antibodies-induced fetal loss [67].

Recently, the excessive activation of complement system at the fetal-maternal interface has been proposed as an additional aPL antibodies-mediated mechanism of placental damage responsible for negative outcome in APS. In pregnant murine model of APS, Girardi et al. demonstrated that aPL antibodies, preferentially targeted at deciduas and placentas, activate the complement system through the classical pathway, leading to generation of potent anaphylatoxins and mediators of effector-cell activation. The recruitment of inflammatory cells accelerates local alternative pathway activation and creates a proinflammatory amplification loop that enhances complement component 3 (C3) activation and deposition, generates additional C3a and C5a and results in further influx of inflammatory cells into the placenta [8].

The pathogenic mechanism of complement-mediated fetal loss induced by aPL antibodies is also supported by the protection that deficiency in complement components confers on the animals, or that follows from in vivo inhibition of complement [68,69]. Hence, the complement system could be a potential therapeutic target in aPL-positive patients.

Interestingly, Girardi and co-workers demonstrated that treatment with heparin prevent complement activation in vivo and protect mice from pregnancy complications induced by aPL antibodies [28]. Such low doses of heparin, lacking anticoagulant effects, inhibited inflammatory responses at the level of leukocyte adhesion and influx and limited tissue injury [70-73] Neither fondaparinux nor hirudin, other anticoagulants without known effects on complement [74], prevented pregnancy loss, demonstrating that anticoagulant therapy gives insufficient protection against APS-associated miscarriage [28].

Moreover, it has been demonstrated that heparin possesses the ability to inhibit lipopolysaccharide-induced proinflammatory cytokines (tumour necrosis factor α, interleukin 6, 8 and 1β) [75], involved in recurrent fetal loss of a murine model of APS [76].

Administration of intravenous immunoglobulin (IVIG) has been proposed as a possible treatment to prevent pregnancy loss in APS. IVIG may act by modulating the effect of cytokines as well as by inhibiting the action of pathological antibodies by either the interaction of the Fc portion of immunoglobulin with Fc receptors or the Fab receptors, or by passively acting as anti-idiotypic. IVIG also modulates the activation and effector functions of B and T lymphocytes, neutralizes pathogenic autoantibodies, and interferes with antigen presentation. Furthermore, the anti-inflammatory effect of IVIG may be due to interaction with the complement system [77].

IVIG have been shown to reduce the number of fetal resorptions in mice in which APS had been induced by immunization with aPL [78]. However, in a multicenter placebo controlled pilot study, the administration to pregnant women with APS of IVIG associated to low-dose aspirin plus heparin did not improve obstetric or neonatal outcomes beyond those achieved with a heparin and low-dose aspirin regimen [79].

Recently, Blank and coworkers demonstrated that anti-anti- β2GPI specific IVIG (sIVIG) are able to improve significantly the pregnancy outcome in BALB/c mice passively infused with anti-β2GPI antibodies. They also observed that incubation of sIVIG restored the anti-β2GPI antibodies-inhibited invasiveness of both JAR cells and human trophoblast cells in vitro. Based on these results, APS sIVIG may be considered as potential specific therapeutic safe compound for developing a treatment for APS patient's early fetal loss [80].

Much research is still needed on the effects and proper indications for IVIG in reproductive failure. However, its prohibitive cost will probably prevent it ever becoming a first-line drug and its place is probably best reserved for severely affected patients who cannot be helped by simpler modes of treatment.

A new potential mechanism of aPL antibodies-mediated fetal loss linking TF and complement activation has been recently proposed. TF, best known as the primary cellular initiator of blood coagulation, also contributes to a variety of biological processes. In particular, TF is involved in inflammation and cell injury processes by interacting with protease-activated receptors (PARs) [81], a subfamily of related G protein-coupled receptors. Complexes of TF-FVIIa and TF-FVIIa-factor Xa (FXa) as well as FXa and thrombin induce pro-inflammatory signals by activating PARs and inducing the expression of TNF-α, interleukins, and adhesion molecules [82–84].

Increased expression of TF on monocytes from patients with APS has been reported [85–87] and in vitro studies support a direct role for aPL antibodies in inducing monocyte TF expression. Indeed, incubation of normal monocytes with IgG from patients with APS or monoclonal aPL antibodies has been shown to induce TF expression and activity in these cells [88–90]. In particular, anti-β2GPI human monoclonal antibodies derived from APS patients enhance monocyte TF mRNA and activity in a β2GPI-dependent fashion [91]. Similarly, aPL antibodies (and specifically anti-β2GPI antibodies) have been shown to induce TF, along with inflammatory cytokines and adhesion molecules, on endothelial cells [92–94].

Ritis et al. reported that complement activation is a fundamental process in determining aPL-induced increase of TF expression on neutrophils. Indeed, in this study the authors showed that complement component C5a induced TF synthesis and expression on neutrophils through interaction with C5a receptor [95].

Based on this finding, Redecha et al. investigated whether TF contributes to aPL antibodies-induced fetal loss in mice and observed that mice treated with aPL antibodies showed strong TF staining throughout the decidua and on embryonic debris [96]. Surprisingly, neither increase in fibrin staining nor thrombi was associated with increased TF staining in deciduas from aPL antibodies-treated mice [96]. Moreover, anticoagulation with hirudin and fondaparinux was not sufficient to prevent pregnancy loss in this model. Neither TF increase nor fetal death was observed in mice deficient in complement component C5a receptor (C5aR) treated with aPL antibodies, demonstrating the importance of C5a-C5aR interaction in TF expression and fetal death in this model of APS. To assess the importance of TF in aPL antibodies-induced fetal injury, Redecha et al. inhibited TF with a monoclonal anti-mTF antibody 1H1 [96]. TF blockade prevented fetal death in aPL antibodies-treated mice also diminishing complement component C3 deposition and neutrophil infiltration in deciduas [96].

Furthermore, Redecha et al. investigated the intracellular pathway of TF complement-mediated activation, observing a 5-fold increase in PAR-2 mRNA expression in neutrophils of aPL antibodies-treated mice when compared to untreated mice or mice treated with control antibodies [97] as well as an increased reactive oxygen species (ROS) production and phago-cytosis in neutrophils from aPL antibodies-treated mice. Interestingly, neutrophils from PAR-2 deficient (PAR-2−/−) mice displayed a dramatic reduction of neutrophil activation in aPL antibodies-treated mice [97]. Also ROS production and phagocytosis were significantly reduced in neutrophils from PAR-2−/−mice treated with aPL antibodies compared with aPL antibodies-treated wild-type mice. Specific monoclonal antibody 10H10 that selectively blocks TF-VIIa signaling through PAR-2, but not antibody 5G9 that only prevents TF procoagulant activity, prevented oxidative burst and increased phagocytosis in mice treated with aPL antibodies [97]. These results are in accordance with the previous observation that anticoagu-lation does not rescue pregnancies in APS [43]. In addition, neutrophils from TF δCT/δCT mice that carry a mutation in the cytoplasmic domain involved in PAR-2 signaling did not show increased oxidative stress and phagocytosis in response to aPL antibodies [97]. This data reinforces the idea that TF-FVIIa signaling is required for neutrophil activation and fetal injury in APS.

The possible application of statins in the prevention of aPL antibodies-related adverse pregnancy outcomes arises from their ability to suppress TF expression in various cell types [98]. Knowing that TF is a crucial mediator in aPL antibodies-induced pregnancy loss and that statins diminish TF expression, Girardi et al. investigated whether statins could prevent pregnancy loss in aPL antibodies-treated mice and demonstrated that simvastatin and pravastatin prevented fetal loss by reducing TF and PAR-2 expression on neutrophils, thus preventing neutrophil activation [99]. aPL antibodies-dependent increase in free radical-mediated lipid peroxidation in decidual tissue was also ameliorated by treatment with statins [99] (Figure 2). These results suggest that statins prevent aPL antibodies-induced neutrophil activation, thus protecting trophoblasts from oxidative damage and rescuing the fetuses. However, given that statins are not major teratogens [100,101] and considering the beneficial effects of statins in animal studies, statins should be considered as a possible treatment for women with aPL antibodies-induced pregnancy complications. Clinical trials are needed to confirm the effectiveness of its application to humans.

Mulla et al. Investigated further mechanisms characterizing the inflammatory process occurring in vitro in trophoblast cells after aPL antibodies binding. Indeed, they demonstrated that anti-β2GPI antibodies trigger an inflammatory response in trophoblast, characterized by increased secretion of IL-8, MCP-1, GRO-α and IL-1β, and that this occurs in a TLR-4/MyD88-dependent manner [102]. At high concentrations, these antibodies also induce caspase-mediated cell death. This was attenuated upon disabling of the MyD88 pathway, suggesting that anti-β2GPI-induced inflammatory mediators compromise trophoblast survival by acting in an autocrine/paracrine manner. Enhanced IL-8, GRO-α and IL-1β secretion also occurred when trophoblast were incubated with antibodies from patients with APS. Heparin attenuated the anti-β2GPI antibody-mediated cell death, and also the pro-inflammatory response, but only at high concentrations [102]. These findings demonstrate that aPL antibodies triggers a

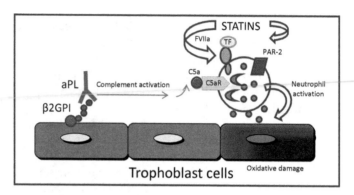

Figure 2. Statins prevent C5a-induced upregulation of TF and PAR2 expression, thereby inhibiting the release of reactive oxygen species and suppressing amplification of complement activation by factors released from neutrophils. Modified from *Girardi G. et al., Journal of Reproductive Immunology 2009* [99].

placental inflammatory response via the TLR-4/MyD88 pathway, which in turn compromises trophoblast survival. Thus, the TLR-4/MyD88 pathway may provide a new therapeutic target to improve pregnancy outcome in APS.

4. Conclusions

Heparin, associated to low dose aspirin, is considered nowadays the gold standard for the prevention of obstetric complications in pregnant women with APS. Yet, heparin therapy administered at subanticoagulant doses has improved pregnancy outcomes in some trials of APS patients [35]. Several studies have proposed different mechanisms of action able to explain the beneficial effect of heparin in preventing adverse pregnancy outcomes associated to APS (Table 2).

↓ aPL antibodies binding to trophoblast cells
↑ Cleavage of β2GPI
↓ Complement activation
↓ Trophoblast cells apoptosis
↑ Trophoblast cells invasiveness and differentiation
↑ HB-EGF expression
↑ Endometrial angiogenesis

Table 2. Heparin mediated mechanisms of placental protection from aPL antibodies.

However, in women with APS and history of obstetric failures, pregnancy complications recur in the 15% of cases despite the therapy.

In the last years new mechanisms of aPL-mediated pregnancy impairment, like inflammation and angiogenesis inhibition, and more specific target therapies have being examined in order to treat more selectively the aPL antibodies-induced placental damage and to ameliorate the reproductive performance of women with APS. Studies on humans are required to verify the safety profile and effectiveness of new therapies proposed.

Author details

Chiara Tersigni, Silvia D'Ippolito and Nicoletta Di Simone

Department of Obstetrics and Gynaecology, Università Cattolica del Sacro Cuore, Rome, Italy

References

[1] Wilson W.A., Gharavi A.E., Koike T., Lockshin M.D., Branch D.W., Piette J.C., Brey R., Derksen R., Harris E.N., Hughes G.R., Triplett D.A. & Khamashta M.A. International consensus statement on preliminary classification criteria for definite antiphospholipid syndrome: report of an international workshop. Arthritis Rheum, Vol. 42, No. 7, (Jul 1999), pp. 1309–1311.

[2] Miyakis S., Lockshin M.D., Atsumi T., Branch D.W., Brey R.L., Cervera R., Derksen R.H., DE Groot P.G., Koike T., Meroni P.L., Reber G., Shoenfeld Y., Tincani A., Vlachoyiannopoulos P.G. & Krilis S.A. International consensus statement on an update of the classification criteria for definite antiphospholipid syndrome (APS). J Thromb Haemost, Vol. 4, No.2, (Feb 2006), pp. 295-306.

[3] Woodhams B.J., Candotti G., Shaw R. & Kernoff P.B. Changes in coagulation and fibrinolysis during pregnancy: evidence of activation of coagulation preceding spontaneous abortion. Thromb Res, Vol. 55, No. 1, (Jul 1989), pp. 99-107.

[4] Chamley L.W. Action of anticardiolipin andantibodies to beta2-glycoprotein-I on trophoblast proliferation as a mechanism for fetal death. Lancet, Vol. 352, No. 9133, (Sep 1998), pp. 1037-1038.

[5] Franklin R.D. & Kutteh W.H. Effects of unfractionated and low molecular weight heparin on antiphospholipid antibody binding in vitro. Obstet Gynecol, Vol. 101, No. 3, (Mar 2003), pp 455–462.

[6] Erkan A., Harrison M.J., Levy R., Peterson M., Petri M., Sammaritano L., Unalp-Arida A., Vilela V., Yazici Y. & Lockshin M.D. Aspirin for primary thrombosis prevention in the antiphospholipid syndrome: a randomized, double-blind, placebo-controlled trial in asymptomatic antiphospholipid antibody-positive individuals. Arthritis Rheum, Vol. 56, No. 7, (Jul. 2007), pp. 2382-2391.

[7]   Holers V.M., Girardi G., Mo L., Guthridge J.M., Molina H., Pierangeli S.S., Espinola R., Xiaowei L.E., Mao D., Vialpando C.G. & Salmon J.E. Complement C3 activation is required for antiphospholipid antibody-induced fetal loss. J Exp Med, Vol. 195, No. 2, (Jan 2002), pp. 211–220.

[8]   Girardi G., Berman J., Redecha P., Spruce L., Thurman J.M., Kraus D., Hollmann T.J., Casali P., Caroll M.C., Wetsel R.A., Lambris J.D., Holers V.M. & Salmon JE. Complement C5a receptors and neutrophils mediate fetal injury in the antiphospholipid syndrome. J Clin Invest, Vol. 112, No. 11, (Dec 2003), pp. 1644–1654.

[9]   Berman J., Girardi G. & Salmon J.E. TNF-α is a critical effector and a target for therapy in antiphospholipid antibody-induced pregnancy loss. J Immunol, Vol. 174, No. 1, (Jan 2005), pp. 485–490.

[10] Miyakis S., Lockshin M.D., Atsumi T., Branch D.W., Brey R.L., Cervera R., Derksen R.H., DE Groot P.G., Koike T., Meroni P.L., Reber G., Shoenfeld Y., Tincani A., Vlachoyiannopoulos P.G. & Krilis S.A. International consensus statement on an update of the classification criteria for definite antiphospholipid syndrome (APS). J Thromb Haemost, Vol. 4, No.2, (Feb 2006), pp. 295-306.

[11] Stirrat G.M. Recurrent miscarriage I: definition and epidemiology. Lancet, Vol. 336, No. 8716, (Sep 1990), pp. 673-675.

[12] Rai R.S., Regan L., Clifford K., Pickering W., Dave M., Mackie I., McNally T. & Cohen H. Antiphospholipid antibodies and ß2-glycoprotein-I in 500 women with recurrent miscarriage: results of a comprehensive screening approach. Hum Reprod, Vol. 10, No. 8, (Aug 1995), pp. 2001-2005.

[13] Yetman D.L. & Kutteh W.H. Antiphospholipid antibody panels and recurrent pregnancy loss: prevalence of anticardiolipin antibodies compared with other antiphospholipid antibodies. Fertil Steril, Vol. 66, No. 4, (Oct 1996), pp. 540-546.

[14] Silver R.M. Fetal death. Obstet Gynecol, Vol. 109, No. 1, (Jan 2007), pp. 153-167.

[15] Smith G.C.S., Crossley J.A., Aitken D.A., Pell J.P., Cameron A.D., Connor J.M. & Dobbie R. First-trimester placentation and the risk of antepartum stillbirth. JAMA, Vol. 292, No. 18, (Nov 2004), pp. 2249–2254.

[16] Oshiro B.T., Silver R.M., Scott J.R., Yu H. & Branch D.W. Antiphospholipid antibodies and fetal death. Obstet Gynecol, Vol. 87, No. 4, (Apr 1996), pp. 489–493.

[17] Clark E.A., Silver R.M. & Branch D.W. Do antiphospholipid antibodies cause preeclampsia and HELLP syndrome? Curr Rheumatol Rep, Vol. 9, No. 3, (Jun 2007), pp. 219-225.

[18] Vora S., Shetty S., Salvi V., SatoskarP. & Ghosh K. Thrombophilia and unexplained loss in Indian patients. Natl Med J India, Vol. 21, No. 3, (Jun 2008), pp. 116-119.

[19] Galli M., Luciani D., Bertolini G. & Barbui T. Anti-beta 2-glycoprotein I, antipro-thrombin antibodies, and the risk of thrombosis in the antiphospholipid syndrome. Blood, 2003, Vol. 102, No. 8, (Oct 2003), pp. 2717-2723.

[20] Rand, J.H., Wu X.X., Quinn A.S. & Taatjes D.J. The annexin A5-mediated pathogenic mechanism in the antiphospholipid syndrome: role in pregnancy losses and throm-bosis. Lupus, Vol. 19, No. 4, (Apr 2010), pp. 460–469.

[21] Pierangeli S.S., Chen P.P., Raschi E., Scurati S., Grossi C., Borghi M.O., Palomo I., Harris E.N. & Meroni P.L. Antiphospholipid antibodies and the antiphospholipid syndrome: pathogenic mechanisms. Semin Thromb Hemost, Vol. 34, No.3, (Apr 2008), pp. 236-250.

[22] Pierangeli S.S., Chen P.P. & González E.B. Antiphospholipid antibodies and the anti-phospholipid syndrome: an update on treatment and pathogenic mechanisms. Curr Opin Hematol, Vol. 13, No. 5, (Sep 2006), pp. 366-375.

[23] Lopez-Pedrera C., Cuadrado M.J., Herández V., Buendïa P., Aguirre M.A., Barbarroja N., Torres L.A., Villalba J.M., Velasco F. & Khamashta M. Proteomic analysis in mon-ocytes of antiphospholipid syndrome patients: Deregulation of proteins related to the development of thrombosis. Arthritis Rheum, Vol. 58, No. 9, (Sep 2008), pp. 2835–2844.

[24] Montiel-Manzano G., Romay-Penabad Z., Papalardo de Martínez E., Meillon-García L.A., García-Latorre E., Reyes-Maldonado E. & Pierangeli S.S. In vivo effects of an in-hibitor of nuclear factor-kappa B on thrombogenic properties of antiphospholipid an-tibodies. Ann N Y Acad Sci, No. 1108, (Jun 2007), pp. 540-553.

[25] Vega-Ostertag M., Casper K., Swerlick R., Ferrara D., Harris E.N. & Pierangeli SS. (2005). Involvement of p38 MAPK in the up-regulation of tissue factor on endothelial cells by antiphospholipid antibodies. Arthritis Rheum, Vol. 52, No. 5, (May 2005), pp. 1545-1554.

[26] de Groot P.G. & Derksen R.H. Pathophysiology of the antiphospholipid syndrome. J Thromb Haemost, Vol. 3, No. 8, (Aug 2005), pp. 1854-1860.

[27] Pierangeli S.S., Girardi G., Vega-Ostertag M., Liu X., Espinola R.G. & Salmon J. Re-quirement of activation of complement C3 and C5 for antiphospholipid antibody mediated thrombophilia. Arthritis Rheum, Vol. 52, No.7, (Jul 2005), pp. 2120-2124.

[28] Girardi G., Redecha P. & Salmon J.E. Heparin prevents antiphospholipid antibody-induced fetal loss by inhibiting complement activation. Nat Med, Vol. 10, No.11, (Nov 2004), pp. 1222-1226.

[29] Meroni P.L., Borghi M.O., Raschi E., Ventura D., Sarzi Puttini P.C., Atzeni F., Lonati L., Parati G., Tincani A., Mari D. & Tedesco F. Inflammatory response and the endo-thelium. Thromb Res, Vol. 114, No.5-6, (2004), pp. 329-334.

[30] Ruiz-Irastorza G., Crowther M., Branch W. & Khamashta M.A. Antiphospholipid syndrome. Lancet, Vol. 76, No. 9751, (Oct 2010), pp. 1498-1509.

[31] Peaceman, A.M. & Rehnberg, K.A. The effect of immunoglobulin G fractions from patients with lupus anticoagulant on placental prostacyclin and thromboxane production. Am J Obstet Gynecol, Vol. 169, No. 6, (Dec 1993), pp. 1403–1406.

[32] Nayar R. & Lage J.M. Placental changes in a first trimester missed abortion in maternal systemic lupus erythematosus with antiphospholipid syndrome; a case report and review of the literature. Hum Pathol, Vol. 27, No. 2, (Feb 1996), pp. 201–206.

[33] Rand, J.H., Wu X.X., Guller S., Gil J., Guha A., Scher J. & Lockwood C.J. Reduction of annexin-V (placental anticoagulant protein-I) on placental villi of women with antiphospholipid antibodies and recurrent spontaneous abortion. Am J Obstet Gynecol, Vol. 171, No. 6, (Dec 1994), pp. 1566–1572.

[34] Horbach D.A., van Oort E., Lisman T., Meijers J.C., Derksen R.H. & de Groot P.G. Beta2-glycoprotein I is proteolytically cleaved in vivo upon activation of fibrinolysis. Thromb Haemost, Vol. 81, No. 1, (Jan 1999), pp. 87-95.

[35] Derksen R.H., Khamasthta M.A. & Branch D.W. Management of the obstetric antiphospholipid syndrome. Arthritis Rheum, Vol., No. 4, (Apr 2004), pp. 1028–1039.

[36] Out H.J., Kooijman C.D., Bruinse H.W. & Derksen R.H. Histopathological finding from patient with intrauterine fetal death and antiphospholipid antibodies. Eur J Obstet Gynecol, Vol. 41, No. 3, (Oct 1991), pp. 179-186.

[37] Park A.L. (2006). Placental pathology in antiphospholipid syndrome, In: Hughes' Syndrome, Khamashta M. A. pp. 362–374, Springer-Verlag, London.

[38] Meroni P.L., Tedesco F., Locati M., Vecchi A., Di Simone N., Acaia B., Pierangeli S.S. & Borghi M.O. Anti-phospholipid antibody mediated fetal loss: still an open question from a pathogenic point of view. Lupus, Vol. 19, No.4, (Apr 2010), pp. 453-456.

[39] Di Simone N., Meroni P.L., de Papa N., Raschi E., Caliandro D., De Carolis C.S., Khamashta M.A., Atsumi T., Hughes G.R., Balestrieri G., Tincani A., Casali P. & Caruso A. Antiphospholipid antibodies affect trophoblast gonadotropin secretion and invasiveness by binding directly and through adhered beta2-glycoprotein I. Arthritis Rheum, Vol. 43, No. 1, (Jan 2000), pp. 140-150.

[40] Katsuragawa H., Kanzaki H., Inoue T., Hirano T., Mori T. & Rote N.S. Monoclonal antibody against phosphatidylserine inhibits in vitro human trophoblastic hormone production and invasion. Biol Reprod, Vol. 56, No. 1, (Jan 1997), pp. 50–58.

[41] Rote N.S., Vogt E., DeVere G., Obringer A.R. & Ng A.K. The role of placental trophoblast in the pathophysiology of the antiphospholipid antibody syndrome. Am J Reprod Immunol, Vol. 39, No. 2, (Feb 1998), pp. 125-136.

[42] Wang S.X., Sun Y.T. & Sui S.F. Membrane-induced conformational change in human apolipoprotein. H Biochem J, Vol. 348, (May 2000), pp. 103–106.

[43] Lyden T.W., Vogt E., Ng A.K., Johnson P.M. & Rote N.S. Monoclonal antiphospholipid antibody reactivity against human placental trophoblast. J Reprod Immunol, Vol. 22, No. 1, (Jun 1992), pp. 1-14.

[44] Guerin J., Sheng Y., Reddel S., Iverson G.M., Chapman M.G. & Krilis S.A. Heparin inhibits the binding of beta 2-glycoprotein I to phospholipids and promotes the plasmin-mediated inactivation of this blood protein. Elucidation of the consequences of the two biological events in patients with the anti-phospholipid syndrome. J Biol Chem, Vol. 277, No. 4, (Jan 2002), pp.2644-2649.

[45] Di Simone N., Ferrazzani S., Castellani R., De Carolis S., Mancuso S. & Caruso A. Heparin and low dose aspirin restore placental human chorionic gonadotrophin secretion abolished by antiphospholipid antibody-containing sera. Hum Reprod, Vol. 12, No. 9, (Sep 1997), pp. 2061-2065.

[46] Di Simone N., Caliandro D., Castellani R., Ferrazzani S., De Carolis S. & Caruso A. Low-molecular weight heparin restores in-vitro trophoblast invasiveness and differentiation in presence of immunoglobulin G fractions obtained from patients with antiphospholipid syndrome. Hum Reprod, Vol. 14, No. 2, (Feb1999), pp. 489-495.

[47] Raab G. & Klagsbrun M. Heparin binding EGF growth factor. Biochim Biophys Acta, Vol. 1333, No. 3, (Dec 1997), pp. 179–99.

[48] Iwamoto R. & Mekada E. Heparin-binding EGF-like growth factor: a juxtacrine growth factor. Cytokine Growth Factor Rev, Vol. 11, No. 4, (Dec 2000), pp. 335-344.

[49] Martin K.L., Barlow D.H. & Sargent I.L. Heparin-binding epidermal growth factor significantly improves human blastocyst development and hatching in serum-free medium. Hum Reprod, Vol. 13, No. 6, (Jun 1998), pp. 1645-1652.

[50] Wang J., Mayernik L., Schultz J.F. & Armant D.R. Acceleration of trophoblast differentiation by heparinbinding EGF-like growth factor is dependent on the stage-specific activation of calcium influx by ErbB receptors in developing mouse blastocysts. Development, Vol. 127, No. 1, (Jan 2000), pp. 33–44.

[51] Paria B.C., Ma W., Tan J., Raja S., Das S.K., Dey S.K. & Hogan B.L. Cellular and molecular responses of the uterus to embryo implantation can be elicited by locally applied growth factors. Proc Natl Acad Sci U S A, Vol. 98, No. 3, (Jan 2001), pp. 1047-1052.

[52] Leach R.E., Khalifa R., Ramirez N.D., Das S.K., Wang J., Dey S.K., Romero R. & Armant D.R. Multiple roles for heparin-binding epidermal growth factor-like growth factor are suggested by its cell-specific expression during the human endometrial cycle and early placentation. J Clin Endocrinol Metab, Vol. 84, No. 9, (Sep 1999), pp. 3355–63.

[53] Leach R.E., Romero R., Kim Y.M., Chaiworapongsa T., Kilburn B., Das S.K., Dey S.K., Johnson A., Qureshi F., Jacques S. & Armant D.R. Pre-eclampsia and expression of heparin-binding EGF-like growth factor. Lancet, Vol. 360, No. 9341, (Oct 2002), pp. 1215-1219.

[54] Di Simone N., Marana R., Castellani R., Di Nicuolo F., D'Alessio M.C., Raschi E., Borghi M.O., Chen P.P., Sanguinetti M., Caruso A. & Meroni P.L. Decreased expression of heparin-binding epidermal growth factor-like growth factor as a newly identified pathogenic mechanism of antiphospholipid-mediated defective placentation. Arthritis Rheum, Vol. 62, No. 5, (May 2010), pp. 1504-1512.

[55] Di Simone N., Di Nicuolo F., D'Ippolito S., Castellani R., Tersigni C., Caruso A., Meroni P. & Marana R. Antiphospholipid antibodies affect human endometrial angiogenesis. Biol Reprod, Vol. 83, No. 2, (Aug 2010), pp. 212-219.

[56] D'Ippolito S., Marana R., Di Nicuolo F., Castellani R., Veglia M., Stinson J., Scambia G. & Di Simone N. Effect of Low Molecular Weight Heparins (LMWHs) on antiphospholipid Antibodies (aPL)-mediated inhibition of endometrial angiogenesis. PLoS One, Vol. 7, No. 1, (Jan 2012), e29660.

[57] Kolyada A., Lee C.J., De Biasio A. & and Beglova N. A novel dimeric inhibitor targeting Beta2GPI in Beta2GPI/antibody complexes implicated in antiphospholipid syndrome. PLoS One, Vol. 5, No. 12, (Dec 2010), e15345.

[58] Ostertag M.V., Liu X., Henderson V. & Pierangeli S.S. A peptide that mimics the Vth region of beta–2–glycoprotein I reverses antiphospholipid–mediated thrombosis in mice. Lupus, Vol. 15, No. 6, (2006), pp. 358–365.

[59] Martinez de la Torre Y., Pregnolato F., D'Amelio F., Grossi C., Di Simone N., Pasqualini F., Nebuloni M., Chen P., Pierangeli S., Bassani N., Ambrogi F., Borghi M.O., Vecchi A., Locati M. & Meroni P.L. Anti–phospholipid induced murine fetal loss: novel protective effect of a peptide targeting the β2 glycoprotein I phospholipid–binding site. Implications for human fetal loss. J Autoimmun, Vol. 38, No. 2-3, (May 2012), pp. 209–215.

[60] Gharavi A.E., Pierangeli S.S., Espinola R.G., Liu.X., Colden-Stanfield M. & Harris E.N. Antiphospholipid antibodies induced in mice by immunization with a cytomegalovirus–derived peptide cause thrombosis and activation of endothelial cells in vivo. Arthritis Rheum, Vol. 46, No. 2, (Feb. 2002), pp. 545–552.

[61] Gharavi A.E., Vega–Ostertag M., Espinola R.G., Liu X., Cole L., Cox N.T., Romagnoli P., Labat K. & Pierangeli S.S.. Intrauterine fetal death in mice caused by cytomegalovirus derived peptide induced aPL antibodies. Lupus, Vol. 13, No. 1, (2004), pp. 17–23.

[62] Del Papa N., Sheng Y.H., Raschi E., Kandiah D.A., Khamashta M.A., Atsumi T., Hughes G.R., Ichikawa K., Koike T., Balestrieri G., Krilis S.A. & Meroni P.L. Human beta 2–glycoprotein I binds to endothelial cells through a cluster of lysine residues

that are critical for anionic phospholipid binding and offers epitopes for anti–beta 2–glycoprotein I antibodies. J Immunol, Vol. 160, No. 11, (Jun 1998), pp. 5572–5578.

[63] Di Simone N., Raschi E., Testoni C., Castellani R., D'Asta M., Shi T., Krilis S.A., Caruso A. & Meroni P.L. Pathogenic role of anti–ß2–glycoprotein I antibodies in antiphospholipid associated fetal loss: characterization of ß2–glycoprotein I binding to trophoblast cells and functional effects of anti–ß2–glycoprotein I antibodies in vitro. Ann Rheum Dis, Vol. 64, No. 3., (Mar 2005), pp. 462–467.

[64] Peaceman A.M & Rehnberg K.A. The effect of immunoglobulin G fractions from patients with lupus anticoagulant on placental prostacyclin and thromboxane production. Am J Obstet Gynecol, Vol. 169, No. 6, (Dec 1993), pp. 1403–1406.

[65] Nayar R. & Lage J.M. Placental changes in a first trimester missed abortion in maternal systemic lupus erythematosus with antiphospholipid syndrome; a case report and review of the literature. Hum Pathol, Vol. 27, No. 2, (Feb 1996), pp. 201–206.

[66] Di Simone N., D'Ippolito S., Marana R., Di Nicuolo F., Castellani R., Pierangeli S.S., Chen P.P., Tersigni C., Scambia G. & Meroni P.L. Antiphospholipid Antibodies Affect Human Endometrial Angiogenesis: protective effect of a synthetic peptide (TIFI) mimicking the phospholipid binding site of β2glycoprotein I. Am J Reprod Immunol, (May 2013) (in press).

[67] Chaouat G. The Th1/Th2 paradigm: still important in pregnancy? Semin Immunopathol, Vol. 29, No. 2, (Jun 2007), pp. 95–113.

[68] Thurman, J.M., Kraus D.M., Girardi G., Hourcade D., Kang H.J., Royer P.A., Mitchell L.M., Giclas P.C., Salmon J., Gilkeson G. & Holers V.M. A novel inhibitor of the alternative complement pathway prevents antiphospholipid antibody-induced pregnancy loss in mice. Mol Immunol, Vol. 42, No. 1, (Jan 2005), pp. 87–97.

[69] Girardi G., Yarilin D., Thurman J.M., Holers V.M. & Salmon J.E. Complement activation induces dysregulation of angiogenic factors and causes fetal rejection and growth restriction. J Exp Med, Vol. 203, No. 9, (Sep 2006), pp. 2165–2175.

[70] Friedrichs G.S., Kilgore K.S., Manley P.J., Gralinsky M.R. & Lucchesi B.R. Effect of heparin and N-acetyl heparin on ischemia/reperfusion-induced alterations in myocardial function in the rabbit isolated heart. Circ Res, Vol. 75, No. 4, (Oct 1994), pp. 701-710.

[71] Koenig A., Norgard-Sumnicht K., Lindhardt R. & Varki A. Differential interactions of heparin and heparan sulfate glycosaminoglycans with the selectins. Implications for the use of unfractionated and low molecular weight heparins as therapeutic agents. J Clin Invest, Vol. 101, No. 4, (Feb 1998), pp. 877-889.

[72] Wang L., Brown J.R., Varki A. & Esko J.D. Heparin's anti-inflammatory effects require glucosamine 6-O-sulfation and are mediated by blockade of L- and P- selectins. J Clin Invest, Vol. 110, No. 1, (Jul 2002), pp. 127-136.

[73] Rops A.L., van der Vlag J., Lensen F.J., Wijnhoven T.J., van den Heuvel L.P., van Kup-pevelt T.H. & Berden J.H. Heparan sulphate proteoglycans in glomerular inflamma-tion. Kidney Int, Vol. 65, No. 3, (Mar 2004), pp. 768-785.

[74] Mollnes T.E., Brekke O.L., Fung M., Fure H., Christiansen D., Berseth G., Videm V., Lappegard K.T., Kökl J. &Lambris J.D. Essential role of the C5a receptor in E coli-in-duced oxidative burst and phagocytosis revealed by a novel lepirudin-based human whole blood model of inflammation. Blood, Vol. 100, No. 5, (Sep 2002), pp. 1869-1877.

[75] Hochart H., Jenkins P.V., Smith O.P. & White B. Low-molecular weight and unfrac-tionated heparins induce a downregulation of inflammation: decreased levels of proinflammatory cytokines and nuclear factor-kappaB in LPS-stimulated human monocytes. Br J Haematol, Vol. 133, No. 1, (Apr 2006), pp. 62-67.

[76] Berman J., Girardi G. & Salmon J.E. TNF-alpha is a critical effector and a target for therapy in antiphospholipid antibody-induced pregnancy loss. J Immunol, Vol. 174, No. 1, (Jan 2005), pp. 485-490.

[77] Carp H.J.A. Intravenous Immunoglobulin: Effect on Infertility and Recurrent Preg-nancy Loss. IMAJ, Vol. 12, No. 9, (Dec 2007), pp. 877–880.

[78] Bakimer R., Gilburd B., Zurgil N. & Shoenfeld Y. The effect of intravenous gamma-globulin on the induction of experimental antiphospholipid syndrome. Clin Immu-nol Immunopathol, Vol. 69, No. 1, (Oct 1993), pp. 97–102.

[79] Branch D.W., Peaceman A.M., Druzin M., Silver R.K., El-Sayed Y., Silver R.M., Esplin M.S., Spinnato J. & Harger J. A multicenter, placebo-controlled pilot study of intrave-nous immune globulin treatment of antiphospholipid syndrome during pregnancy. The Pregnancy Loss Study Group. Am J Obstet Gynecol, Vol. 182, No. 1, (Jan 2000), pp. 122–127.

[80] Blank M., Anafi L., Zandman-Goddard G., Krause I., Goldman S., Shalev E., Cervera R., Font J., Fridkin M., Thiesen H.J. & Shoenfeld Y. The efficacy of specific IVIG anti-idiotypic antibodies in antiphospholipid syndrome (APS): trophoblast invasiveness and APS animal model. International Immunology, Vol. 19, No. 7, (Jul 2007), pp. 857–865.

[81] Camerer E., Huang W. & Coughlin S.R. Tissue factor and factor X-dependent activa-tion of ptotease-activated receptor 2 by factor VIIa. Proc Natl Acad Sci USA, Vol. 97, No. 10, (May 2000), pp. 5255-5260.

[82] Ruf W., Dorfleutner A. & Riewald M. Specificity of coagulation factor signaling. J Thromb Haemost, Vol. 1, No. 7, (Jul 2003), pp. 1495–1503.

[83] Mueller B.M., Reisfeld R.A., Edgington T.S. & Ruf W. Expression of tissue factor by melanoma cells promotes efficient hematogenous metastasis. Proc Natl Acad Sci USA, Vol. 89, No. 24, (Dec1992), pp. 1–6.

[84] Cuadrado M.J., López-Pedrera C., Khamashta M.A. Camps M.T., Tinahones F., Torres A., Hughes G.R. & Velasco F. Thrombosis in primary antiphospholipid syndrome: a pivotal role for monocyte tissue factor expression. Arthritis Rheum, Vol. 40, No. 5 (May 1997), pp. 834–841.

[85] Dobado-Berrios P.M., Lopez-Pedrera C., Velasco F., Aguirre M.A., Torres A. & Cuadrado M.J. Increased levels of tissue factor mRNA in mononuclear blood cells of patients with primary antiphospholipid syndrome. Thromb Haemost, Vol. 82, No. 6, (Dec 1999), pp.1578–1582.

[86] Reverter J.C., Tassies D., Font J., Monteagudo J., Escolar J., Ingelmo M. & Ordinas A. Hypercoagulable state in patients with antiphospholipid syndrome is related to high induced tissue factor expression on monocytes and to low free protein S. Arterioscler Thromb Vasc Biol, Vol. 16, No. 11, (Nov 1996), pp. 1319–1326.

[87] Nojima J., Masuda Y., Iwatani Y., Suehisa E., Futsukaichi Y., Kuratsune H., Watanabe Y., Takano T., Hidaka Y., Kanakura Y. Tissue factor expression on monocytes induced by anti-phospholipid antibodies as a strong risk factor for thromboembolic complications in SLE patients. Biochem Biophys Res Commun, Vol. 365, No. 1 (Jan 2008), pp. 195–200.

[88] Amengual O., Atsumi T., Khamashta M.A. & Hughes G.R.V. The role of the tissue factor pathway in the hypercoagulable state in patients with the antiphospholipid syndrome. Thromb Haemost, Vol. 79, No. 2, (Feb 1998), pp. 276–281.

[89] Zhou H., Walberg A.S. & Roubey R.A.S. Characterization of monocyte tissue factor activity induced by IgG antiphospholipid antibodies and inhibition by dilazep. Blood, Vol. 104, No. 8, (Oct 2004), pp. 2353–2358.

[90] Roubey R.A., Pratt C.W., Buyon J.P. & Winfield J.B. Lupus anticoagulant activity of autoimmune antiphospholipid antibodies is dependent upon beta 2-glycoprotein I. J Clin Invest, Vol. 90, No. 3, (Sep 1992), pp. 1100–1104.

[91] Vega-Ostertag M., Casper K., Swerlick R., Ferrara D., Harris E.N. & Pierangeli S.S. Involvement of p38 MAPK in the upregulation of tissue factor on endothelial cells by antiphospholipid antibodies. Arthritis Rheum, Vol. 52, No. 5, (May 2005), pp. 1545–1554.

[92] Lopez-Pedrera C., Buendia P., Barbarroja N., Siendones E., Velasco F. & Cuadrado M.J. Antiphospholipid-mediated thrombosis: interplay between anticardiolipin antibodies and vascular cells. Clin Appl Thromb Hemost, Vol. 12, No. 1, (Jan 2006), pp. 41–45.

[93] Kornberg A., Renaudineau Y., Blank M., Youinou P. & Sheffield Y. Anti-beta2-glycoprotein I antibodies and anti-endothelial cell antibodies induce tissue factor in endothelial cells. Isr Med Assoc J, Vol. 2, (Jul 2000), pp.27–31.

[94] Vega-Ostertag M.E., Ferrara D.E., Romay-Penabad Z., Liu X., Taylor W.R., Colden-Stanfield M. & Pierangeli S.S. Role of p38 mutagen-activated protein kinas in anti-

phospholipid antibodymediated thrombosis and endothelial cell activation. J Thromb Haemost, Vol. 5, No. 9, (Sep 2007), pp.1828–1834.

[95] Ritis K., Doumas M., Mastellos D., Micheli A., Glaglis S., Magotti P., Rafail S., Kartalis G., Sideras P. & Lambris J.D. A novel C5a receptor-tissue factor cross-talk in neutrophils links innate immunity to coagulation pathways. J Immunol, Vol. 177, No. 7, (Oct 2006), pp. 4794–4802.

[96] Redecha P., Tilley R., Tencati M., Samon J.E., Kirchhofer D., Mackman N. & Girardi G. Tissue factor: a link between C5a and neutrophil activation in antiphospholipid antibody induced fetal injury. Blood, Vol. 110, No. 7, (Oct 2007), pp. 2423–2431.

[97] Redecha P., Franzke C.W., Ruf W., Mackman N. & Girardi G. Neutrophil activation by the tissue factor/Factor VIIa/PAR2 axis mediates fetal death in a mouse model of antiphospholipid syndrome. J Clin Invest, Vol. 118, No. 10, (Oct 2008), pp. 3453–3461.

[98] Kunieda Y., Nakagawa K., Nishimura H., Kato H., Ukimura N., Yano S., Kawano H., Kimura S., Nakagawa M. &Tsuji H. HMG CoA reductase inhibitor suppresses the expression of tissue factor and plasminogen activator inhibitor-1 induced by angiotensin II in cultured rat aortic endothelial cells. Thromb Res, Vol. 110, No. 4, (Jun 2003), pp. 227–234.

[99] Girardi G. Pravastatin prevents miscarriages in antiphospholipid antibody-treated mice. Journal Reprod Immunol, Vol. 82, No. 2, (Nov. 2009), pp. 126–131.

[100] Pollack P.S., Shields K.E., Burnett D.M., Osborne M.J., Cunningham M.L. & Stepanavage M.E. Pregnancy outcomes after maternal exposure to simvastatin and lovastatin. Birth Defects Res A Clin Mol Teratol, Vol. 73, No. 11, (Nov 2005), pp.888–896.

[101] Edison R.J. & Muenke M. Mechanistic and epidemiologic considerations in the evaluation of adverse birth outcomes following gestational exposure to statins. Am J Med Genet A, Vol. 131, No. 3, (Dec 2004), pp. 230–231.

[102] Mulla M.J., Brosens J.J., Chamley L.W., Giles I., Pericleous C., Rahman A., Joyce S.K., Panda B., Paidas M.J. & Abrahams V.M. Antiphospholipid antibodies induce a proinflammatory response in first trimester trophoblast via the TLR4/MyD88 pathway. Am J Reprod Immunol, Vol. 62, No. 2, (Aug 2009), pp. 96-111.

Permissions

The contributors of this book come from diverse backgrounds, making this book a truly international effort. This book will bring forth new frontiers with its revolutionizing research information and detailed analysis of the nascent developments around the world.

We would like to thank Petar Ivanov, MD, PhD, for lending his expertise to make the book truly unique. He has played a crucial role in the development of this book. Without his invaluable contribution this book wouldn't have been possible. He has made vital efforts to compile up to date information on the varied aspects of this subject to make this book a valuable addition to the collection of many professionals and students.

This book was conceptualized with the vision of imparting up-to-date information and advanced data in this field. To ensure the same, a matchless editorial board was set up. Every individual on the board went through rigorous rounds of assessment to prove their worth. After which they invested a large part of their time researching and compiling the most relevant data for our readers. Conferences and sessions were held from time to time between the editorial board and the contributing authors to present the data in the most comprehensible form. The editorial team has worked tirelessly to provide valuable and valid information to help people across the globe.

Every chapter published in this book has been scrutinized by our experts. Their significance has been extensively debated. The topics covered herein carry significant findings which will fuel the growth of the discipline. They may even be implemented as practical applications or may be referred to as a beginning point for another development. Chapters in this book were first published by InTech; hereby published with permission under the Creative Commons Attribution License or equivalent.

The editorial board has been involved in producing this book since its inception. They have spent rigorous hours researching and exploring the diverse topics which have resulted in the successful publishing of this book. They have passed on their knowledge of decades through this book. To expedite this challenging task, the publisher supported the team at every step. A small team of assistant editors was also appointed to further simplify the editing procedure and attain best results for the readers.

Our editorial team has been hand-picked from every corner of the world. Their multi-ethnicity adds dynamic inputs to the discussions which result in innovative outcomes. These outcomes are then further discussed with the researchers and contributors who give their valuable feedback and opinion regarding the same. The feedback is then collaborated with the researches and they are edited in a comprehensive manner to aid the understanding of the subject.

Apart from the editorial board, the designing team has also invested a significant amount of their time in understanding the subject and creating the most relevant covers. They scrutinized every image to scout for the most suitable representation of the subject and create an appropriate cover for the book.

The publishing team has been involved in this book since its early stages. They were actively engaged in every process, be it collecting the data, connecting with the contributors or procuring relevant information. The team has been an ardent support to the editorial, designing and production team. Their endless efforts to recruit the best for this project, has resulted in the accomplishment of this book. They are a veteran in the field of academics and their pool of knowledge is as vast as their experience in printing. Their expertise and guidance has proved useful at every step. Their uncompromising quality standards have made this book an exceptional effort. Their encouragement from time to time has been an inspiration for everyone.

The publisher and the editorial board hope that this book will prove to be a valuable piece of knowledge for researchers, students, practitioners and scholars across the globe.

List of Contributors

Ludek Slavik
Hemato-oncology Clinic, Faculty of Medicine and Dentistry Palacky University Olomouc, Czech Republic

Ricardo Barini, Joyce Annichino-Bizzache, Egle Couto, Marcelo Luis Nomura and Isabela Nelly Machado
Faculdade de Ciências Médicas UNICAMP, SP, Brazil

P. Ivanov
Clinical Institute for Reproductive Medicine, Pleven, Bulgaria
Department of Biochemistry, Medical University of Pleven, Bulgaria

Tsv. Tsvyatkovska
Department of Biochemistry, Medical University of Pleven, Bulgaria

Ivana Novaković and Nela Maksimović
Faculty of Medicine, University of Belgrade, Belgrade, Serbia

Dragana Cvetković
Faculty of Biology, University of Belgrade, Belgrade, Serbia

Patricia J. Dhar and Robert J. Sokol
Wayne State University School of Medicine, Departments of Internal Medicine and Obstetrics & Gynecology, Division of Rheumatology, C.S. Mott Center for Human Growth and Development, Detroit, Michigan, USA

Sl. Tomov
Deparment of Oncogynecology, Medical University of Pleven, Pleven, Bulgaria

E. Konova
Clinical Institute for Reproductive Medicine, Pleven, Bulgaria
Center of Clinical Immunology, University Hospital of Pleven, Pleven, Bulgaria

R. Komsa-Penkova
Department of Biochemistry, Medical University of Pleven, Pleven, Bulgaria

Chiara Tersigni, Silvia D'Ippolito and Nicoletta Di Simone
Department of Obstetrics and Gynaecology, Università Cattolica del Sacro Cuore, Rome, Italy

.

Printed in the USA
CPSIA information can be obtained
at www.ICGtesting.com
JSHW011341221024
72173JS00003B/186